Adapting Yoga for
People Living with Cancer

of related interest

Yoga for a Happy Back
A Teacher's Guide to Spinal Health through Yoga Therapy
Rachel Krentzman, PT, E-RYT
Foreword by Aadil Palkhivala
ISBN 978 1 84819 271 3
eISBN 978 0 85701 253 1

The Yoga Teacher Mentor
A Reflective Guide to Holding Spaces, Maintain-
ing Boundaries, and Creating Inclusive Classes
Jess Glenny
Foreword by Norman Blair
ISBN 978 1 78775 126 2
eISBN 978 1 78775 127 9

Aromatherapy, Massage and Relaxation in Cancer Care
An Integrative Resource for Practitioners
Edited by Ann Carter and Dr Peter A. Mackereth
ISBN 978 1 84819 281 2
eISBN 978 0 85701 228 9

Combining Touch and Relaxation Skills for Cancer Care
The HEARTS Process
Ann Carter
ISBN 978 1 84819 352 9
eISBN 978 0 85701 311 8

ADAPTING YOGA FOR PEOPLE LIVING WITH CANCER

JUDE MILLS

FOREWORD BY CHARLOTTE WATTS

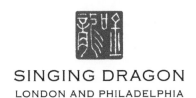

SINGING DRAGON

LONDON AND PHILADELPHIA

First published in Great Britain in 2021 by Singing Dragon,
an imprint of Jessica Kingsley Publishers
An Hachette Company

1

Copyright © Jude Mills 2021

The right of Jude Mills to be identified as the Author of the Work has been asserted
by her in accordance with the Copyright, Designs and Patents Act 1988.

Foreword copyright © Charlotte Watts 2021

Front cover image source: Shutterstock®.

Disclaimer: The information contained in this book is not intended to replace
the services of trained medical professionals or to be a substitute for medical
advice. The complementary therapy described in this book may not be suitable for
everyone to follow. You are advised to consult a doctor before embarking on any
complementary therapy programme and on any matters relating to your health, and
in particular on any matters that may require diagnosis or medical attention.

A CIP catalogue record for this title is available from the
British Library and the Library of Congress

ISBN 978 1 78775 650 2
eISBN 978 1 78775 651 9

Printed and bound in Great Britain by CPI Group

Jessica Kingsley Publishers' policy is to use papers that are natural, renewable
and recyclable products and made from wood grown in sustainable
forests. The logging and manufacturing processes are expected to conform
to the environmental regulations of the country of origin.

Jessica Kingsley Publishers
Carmelite House
50 Victoria Embankment
London EC4Y 0DZ

www.singingdragon.com

For Richard McKeown

Contents

Foreword

I was very pleased to be asked to write this foreword and to have the opportunity of introducing such a heartfelt, honest and deeply useful body of work. I do not say 'useful' in the sense of solving or fixing an issue – such an ingrained reaction in our goal-oriented society – rather, I mean useful in the sense of meeting a true need for so many.

A diagnosis of cancer represents a greatest fear for so many and is often dominated by the 'what to do' aspect of 'the problem'. People with any life-changing diagnosis (and the 'big C' is right up there of course) can understandably be driven to seek solutions. Beyond the first receipt of bad news and the individual reactions this provokes, lies the potential of a recognition that we are still 'us' – a person *with* a condition, not something *other* identified by its label.

I have dedicated the last 25 years of my life to understanding health through the lenses of yoga and nutritional therapy. As well as teaching and practising these holistic modalities, they have been a route through my own chronic illness and in turn I have supported many through the varied processes of disease states. Those I have supported with cancer – or who have a history of or worry about it – have a multitude of ideas, attitudes and responses. These cannot be reduced to 'the disease'; rather they reflect a culmination of the life they have lived – their fears come to the surface, their doubts move into the foreground and their hopes may come into clarity. The full spectrum of what it is to be human – in the words of Rumi, 'the shame, the grief, the malice' – can come into sharp relief.

All of these journeys have of course been personal and individual and do not come along with any prescribed set of rules, expectations or what is 'right' for the individual. When people with cancer are reduced to 'the condition', there can be little room left for a healthy relationship with self and life. This can sometimes occur within the medicalization that can accompany such a diagnosis. When we may feel we have handed over our power, our voice or a piece of ourselves to the 'experts', the path of yoga offers a cogent somato-emotional (body-mind) route to attend to all of our needs, not just those dictated by a named disease.

True empowerment comes from the deep relationship with all aspects of our selves that can be met through compassionate awareness. That can be a tricky journey to navigate when we may feel the disordered relationship with this body that is our home. Rather than simply a list of 'tools', this book is that compassionate guide; a beacon of coming into a kind and attentive space when an idea of a future path appears to have been knocked off course.

Where a cancer diagnosis can dominate our internal experiences and outer relationships with the world and others, the path of yoga offers many cogent aspects of meeting our responses and adapting as we need, moment-to-moment. In these pages, Jude skilfully offers a navigation back to centre and self, using the Yamas (restraints) and Niyamas (observances) from the eight-limbed path of *Yoga Sutras of Patañjali* as a poetic and creative guide to self-enquiry. This is always the true basis of the self-study (Svadhyaya) of the yoga path, not the louder physical aspect of practice that can in its most connected form create embodiment, but which may also feed into a punitive and pushing relationship with the body via idealised poses and body image.

An approach of loving-kindness can also steer us away from common language of 'battles' and 'fighting' so often brought out in a warrior-spirit against an entity we may want to view as an enemy. Whilst I know many find this phraseology motivating and empowering, I am also wary of adding in another layer of combative and hardening mindsets and attitudes that ripple through body tissues and cells. Examining our relationships with these cycles of psychosocial stressors that ripple through our culture and (shown by a large body of evidence) feed into trauma patterns and inflammation that affect immune expression.

This is not to point a judgement, but rather a call to observe and explore the affects that all forms of language and communication towards ourselves affect our entire mind-body (our psycho-neuro-immunology) – in this book, Jude beautifully uses poetry as the vessel to move towards a dialect not of a battle or a fight, but of curiosity, consciousness and the flowering potential of our awareness and authenticity.

For me, the yoga journey offers a coming home to the body as poetry, not reduced into cold mechanics, but describing an orchestration that is in continual shift, with many colours, textures and flavours. Looking inward towards all these expressions – whether we might deem them 'good' or 'bad' – particularly in the face of something as unwanted as cancer, is the route to agency and freedom. It is not an easy journey, but as Jude courageously guides here, it has the potential to be rich and illuminating.

Charlotte Watts, yoga teacher, nutritional therapist, author of
Yoga Therapy for Digestive Health and *The De-Stress Effect*

Padmasana

I have spoken (as if I knew)
Of their thousand-petalled awakenings,
and their ripe heart-openings.

Of how they are cupped
as symbols of purity
in the hands of Goddesses,
and sat upon by Buddhas.

Of how the tombs of
long-dead princesses,
are graced by carvings
as soft and clean as the
living flesh of
the blossoms they honour.

Of how they bloom, Koan-ready
from the silt and the muck

to open, fragrant, mudless
into a foreign sun. Where
the thousand folds are symbols
for other infinite unfoldings
of consciousness.

But I have never
Seen a lotus flower.

Acknowledgements

My deepest gratitude goes to:

All of the people who have trusted me to guide them with yoga during their experience of living with, and going through treatment for, cancer. They all hold a very special place in my heart. I often learned more from them than they did from me, showing me how to do this work, and helping me to share it with many others.

My Healing Space and Yoga for Cancer students and graduates. They are all out in the world offering this work in many different ways and helping to make many people's lives easier. They have also contributed so much to this journey and to the shape that my courses, and this book, have taken.

My partner Richard, who is my cheerleader, and my proofreader, and at all times a voice of kindness and gentle encouragement. Thanks Rich.

To all my teachers over many years who have contributed to my ever-changing and evolving conversation with yoga.

To my friend and colleague, Jess Glenny, who encouraged me to have this book published, and who made the necessary introductions.

To the wonderful team at Jessica Kingsley Publishers, whose patience, guidance and generously accessible process made it possible for this book to finally make it into print.

To all of you – and those I haven't mentioned – a deep bow.

Introduction

Welcome to *Adapting Yoga for People with Cancer*. This book is for yoga teachers who wish to teach yoga to people who are living with a diagnosis of cancer. It serves as a textbook for those who are studying to become yoga therapists and specialist Yoga for Cancer teachers, and as a learning resource for other yoga teachers who want to feel more confident in adapting the practices of yoga for people with cancer.

In 2010, I had been working in the field of wellbeing for people living with cancer for several years, and was working as a yoga teacher and relaxation therapist for a cancer charity attached to a large oncology centre. A friend and fellow yoga teacher came to me and asked if I could teach her to (in her words) 'Do what you do.' She had her own experience of breast cancer, and felt very called to work with others. It was out of that conversation that the Healing Space course was born. The content of this book arises out of that work: teaching Yoga for Cancer, and teaching other yoga teachers to do the same. It is the result of a lot of research and many hours of practice. However, it comes in the most part from what I have learned from the people who have trusted me with some part of their experience of living with cancer, and coping with the treatments.

It is with joy, but also slight trepidation, that I embark on this project. Both yoga, and the study of cancer, are vast topics that can only be covered in a very general way in such a book. For this reason, I have taken the approach of writing within an ethical framework, using the Yamas and Niyamas of Patañjali's Yoga Sutras as my structure. The poetic interpretations – in Haiku form – of the Sutras are my own. They are poems first and foremost – a writer's indulgence – and they are not direct translations from the Sanskrit. I have some basic understanding of the language, but I am in no way a scholar. Rather, they are interpretations based on my reading of many other translations, and the direct English transliterations of the Sanskrit words. My teacher Mukunda Stiles[1] reignited my study of the Sutras, when, like many a yoga teacher, I had consigned them to the shelf immediately after my initial teacher training. His transliteration of the Sanskrit was my key guide in this exercise.

Using an ethical, rather than a purely practical framework helped me to create a structure wherein we can look at the subject of teaching yoga to people with cancer in a way that safeguards both their safety and our own professional boundaries as teachers. Within this framework are a series of questions for reflection and an invitation to create an ongoing reflective practice as a teacher and practitioner of yoga.

Yama

Yama translates as *restraint*. So essentially, the Yamas are calling for the things that we are invited to avoid, or not do, in order to cultivate a healthy yoga practice. These are:

- Ahimsa: non-harming or non-violence.

- Satya: honesty, truthfulness.

- Asteya: non-stealing.

- Brahmacharya: sexual restraint (often translated as celibacy); essentially this means avoiding the unnecessary dissipation of one's energy.

- Aparigraha: non-grasping, non-possessiveness, non-attachment.

Niyama

Niyama translates as *observances*. So Niyamas are the things that you are invited to observe or cultivate for a yoga practice. These are:

- Saucha: purity, cleanliness, clarity.

- Santosha: contentment, acceptance, satisfaction.

- Tapas: austerity, self-discipline, enthusiasm, commitment.

- Svadhyaya: self-study.

- Ishvara Pranhidana: dedication, devotion or surrender to the divine nature (that which is bigger than yourself).

This is not a 'how to' book, and I am sorry if that is what you were hoping for. There is no system that can teach you how to adapt the practices of yoga for cancer, or any other disease, or indeed, any human being. Yes, it does contain information, and advice, and scientific data, and guidelines for practices, but there are no 'off the shelf' practices. First and foremost, this book is an exploration of yourself as a practitioner of yoga and as a teacher.

In her book *Being with Dying* Roshi Joan Halifax[2] writes, 'Life-threatening illness calls us to a place – metaphorically a desert or mountain peak – where, as we sit, the hard wind of reality strips away all the trappings of life, like so much clothing, makeup, and accessories.'

It is in this place that you are invited on a path of discovery, how to be truly present to another human being – in their vulnerability, distress, pain... In their, and our, full humanness.

CHAPTER ONE

Ahimsa

Practise non-harming.
Cultivate a culture of
wellbeing for all.

I begin with Ahimsa as the starting point for this exploration. Ahimsa translates as non-harming or non-violence. And it is in this spirit of doing no harm that I wish to introduce this work. In the context of this enquiry, this means that I look at ways of creating a safe environment to work with people who are living with cancer, who are essentially vulnerable, physically and emotionally – first, from the perspective of creating a safe, comfortable and appropriate space to work in, including adaptations and ways of 'making do'. Then I focus on the physiological side of cancer, treatments, side effects and considerations for adapting the practice, so that you are equipped with enough knowledge to practise safely. Finally, I look at language and its capacity to harm or to heal.

Why do this work?

▮ QUESTIONS FOR REFLECTION

Why are you here? What has drawn you to this book, and to this work?

Take some time to consider, and make notes in your notebook or practice journal. All of the notes you make in these reflective practices will be useful to come back to as you work your way through the book.

Although it might seem like a strange way to start a conversation about Ahimsa, beginning any exploration with a process of self-enquiry is, I believe, a healthy starting point. I have noticed, in the years of teaching the Healing Space course, that this question is one that can be quite triggering. I have asked it of myself, and been poked by it, many, many times. Perhaps because of this, I believe it is one of the healthiest questions we can ask ourselves in reflective practice. It saves us from our unhealthiest motivations, especially those that could potentially lead to burnout.

I know from my own experience that if I find such a question activating, for whatever reason, then there is probably a good reason to keep asking and answering it until it doesn't trigger me any more. This might sound like a challenge, and in some ways it is. However, in exploring Ahimsa, I also offer the invitation to look at the ways in which we are potentially harming ourselves. In Chapter Three I invite an exploration of some of the possible shadow sides of the urge to want to help that may feed your self-reflection as you begin this work.

No answers are invalid; this process of reflection is not about shaming you or trying to put you off. It is about the deep and necessary process of self-enquiry that the practice of yoga invites us into. In choosing to work with people who are vulnerable, you are entering into a realm that is essentially therapeutic, whether you call it that or not. By inviting exposure to the potential suffering of other human beings, being ready to really understand why you are there is a good, solid ethical foundation on which to build a professional practice.

Yoga and cancer

QUESTION FOR REFLECTION

What do you feel when you hear or read the word 'cancer'?

Make some notes in your notebook or practice journal that you can refer back to as you work through this book.

What is cancer?

For a long time, cancer was a frightening, taboo word, a word that spelled a death sentence to the person who had it and in the minds of those who heard it. And cancer – even just the word – still has the power to instil fear, shame and hopelessness.

Thankfully, treatments and screening methods have come a long way, and many cancers can either be treated effectively (cured) or made liveable with. Cancer, for many, has become a long-term illness, like diabetes or heart disease, something that can be managed so that the person living with it can live a long, productive and pain-free life. Even if someone's life is shortened by cancer, the journey towards dying can be comfortable, compassionate and dignified.

Cancer is slowly losing its taboo. People are much more open to discussing it. But my feeling is that we still have a long way to go. In the UK, more people die from heart disease than lung cancer[3] (the leading cause of deaths from cancer), yet we don't seem to fear heart disease in the same way.

▪ QUESTION FOR REFLECTION
What messages have you heard about cancer? Facts, myths, words, scare stories?

It is perhaps because of the fear associated with a diagnosis of cancer that yoga has such a valuable and beautiful part to play in the complementary and holistic treatment we can offer. Yoga is complementary in that it works alongside conventional medicine, and it is holistic in that it works with the whole person – mind, body and spirit.

This has been a reason – as well as the lack of evidence-based material – for modern medicine to be sceptical about holistic or alternative practices in the past. When you start talking to doctors about energy, for example, they often stop listening, and perhaps understandably so. In this respect, teachers might want to tread lightly. If you want to work alongside the medical profession (and this is the best way to access people living with cancer), then it's best to emphasize the evidence. This is not to throw out the baby with the bath water – yoga is yoga – but in my time working in the healthcare environment I have learned that delicate navigation is generally called for.

Cancer biology

Cancer is not just one disease; cancer is the collective name for a diverse range of illnesses with a diverse range of causes and profiles. There are over 200 types of cancer[4] because there are about 200 different types of cells in the human body, and each one can develop cancer. Some cancers are more common, and some are so rare that you may never hear of them. The four most common cancers, in the UK and worldwide, are breast, lung, bowel and prostate.[5]

Cancer is a disease caused when normal cells in the body begin to change and start to grow in an uncontrolled way, causing a tumour or growth. If the cancer is left untreated, the cancer cells can spread to surrounding tissues or to other organs in the body. When cancer spreads to other organs, this is known as metastasis.

Staging and grading

When someone is diagnosed with cancer, their oncologist will ascertain the stage and/or grade of the cancer in order to decide on the appropriate treatment. There are different systems used, and they can be very complicated, but they are all designed to describe how far the cancer has developed, and how the cancer cells behave compared to normal cells.

TNM staging system

'T' refers to the size of the tumour; it is normally numbered between 1 and 4, where 1 is a small cancer and 4 is large or advanced.

'N' refers to spread to the lymph nodes; it is usually numbered between 0 and 3. A numbering of 0 means there are no cancer cells in the lymph nodes and 3 means that the cancer has been found in more lymph nodes.

'M' refers to metastasis; it is numbered 0 or 1. A numbering of 0 means no metastasis and 1 means that the cancer has spread to another part, or parts, of the body.

Number staging system

This is a commonly used method of staging a cancer; it is normally numbered between 1 and 4. Stage 1 means that the cancer is at an early stage and hasn't spread. Stage 4 means that the cancer has spread, that it has metastasized.

Grading

Grading describes how the cancer cells compare with normal cells. This is normally a grading system between 1 and 3:

- A grade of 1 means that the cancer cells look most similar to normal cells and are growing relatively slowly.

- A grade of 2 means that the cancer cells look less like normal cells, or are more abnormal, and are growing more quickly.

- A grade of 3 means that the cancer cells look very different from normal cells, and may grow more quickly.

Cancer treatments and side effects

People who experience cancer will often be offered surgery, chemotherapy or radiotherapy, and these tend to be the frontline treatments. People with blood cancers such as leukaemia may also receive stem cell transplantation. Most people have heard of chemotherapy and radiotherapy, and often assume that anybody who has cancer will receive these treatments, but this is not necessarily the case.

Other treatments that people may receive include targeted treatments such as biological or hormone therapies. Some people may also receive supportive treatments such as blood transfusion or platelet exchange. Other treatments include pain relief medication, anti-nausea medication, steroids and drugs to treat side effects such as dry skin or fungal infections.

Some people may not receive any treatment other than symptom relief depending on the presentation and progression of their disease. Some people may choose not to have conventional treatment at all, relying instead on alternatives such as complementary therapies and diet. People who have had treatment for cancer often tell me that the worst part is the side effects of the treatments.

Surgery

Surgery is a routine treatment for some cancers where it is possible to remove the diseased tissue. A tumour, lump or area of affected skin may be removed, including some of the tissue surrounding it, or a larger area of tissue, an organ or a body part may need to be surgically removed. Surgery is traumatic to the body and can result in side effects such as pain, tightness, loss of sensation, weakness or impaired range of movement.

Chemotherapy

Chemotherapy is treatment by drugs – administered intravenously or orally – that stops cancer cells reproducing. Because cancer cells are fast growing, and many chemotherapy drugs target these fast-growing cells, other fast-growing cells are also affected. These include hair cells, skin cells, blood cells and the cells of the mucous membranes of the mouth, throat, stomach and digestive tract.

This can cause nausea, vomiting or diarrhoea; tiredness and fatigue; peripheral neuropathy (loss of sensation, tingling or pins and needles in the extremities); hair loss; skin problems such as itching, flaking, rash or burning; mucositis (where the mucous membranes in the mouth or digestive tract become severely inflamed); loss of muscle tone; anaemia; and decrease of immune function.

Radiotherapy

Radiotherapy is treatment by radiation, similar to an X-ray administered externally by machine, or internally by the placement of radioactive implants near the cancer (brachytherapy). Radiotherapy is offered after surgery for some cancers to reduce the risk of recurrence, and before surgery for some cancers to shrink the cancer and make it easier to remove.

Radiation treatment can cause burns to the skin and internal tissues, like very severe sunburn, and people also report that it makes them very tired. It can also cause severe irritation to the bladder or bowel, causing issues with going to the toilet. Overall, people often report symptoms of sleeplessness, extreme fatigue, depression and anxiety, and sometimes even panic.

Stem cell transplantation

Stem cells are blood cells in the earliest stage of development that are made in the bone marrow. Stem cell transplantation is usually offered for the treatment of leukaemia, lymphoma and myeloma if other treatments haven't worked or if there is a high risk of the cancer recurring. It involves storing a person's own stem cells (autologous transplant) and then giving them back after high dose chemotherapy, or receiving stem cells from a donor (allogeneic transplant).

Side effects include lowered immunity and risk of infection, anaemia, nausea and vomiting, sore mouth and problems eating, diarrhoea, hair loss and fatigue.

EXERCISE

Using the many excellent online resources and free publications offered by trusted cancer support organizations, make your own list of the potential side effects of chemotherapy and radiotherapy that might be significant when adapting a yoga practice for someone, or indeed that might be helped by some of the practices of yoga. A list of organizations is included in 'Resources to Inform Your Research' at the end of the book.

Treatment considerations for adapting the practice

▦ QUESTIONS FOR REFLECTION

What are your feelings about adapting yoga for people who are going through cancer treatment? Is there anything that is worrying you?

The following list outlines considerations for adapting the yoga practice that you may encounter when you work with people living with cancer. This list applies in addition to the contraindications that you will already be aware of for the general population engaging in a physical yoga practice, for example, adaptations for high blood pressure.

This list is not exhaustive. Everyone is different, everyone's cancer is different, and everyone's treatment is different. I have listed some of the key issues that you might encounter, but please do consult the literature available from organizations such as the NHS, Macmillan and Cancer Research UK for a more comprehensive understanding of the full range of side effects.

Chemotherapy

- Low immunity: *For this reason, you cannot work with this person if you have an active infection, of any kind – even a cold.*

- Nausea, diarrhoea or constipation.

- Intense fatigue.

- Hair loss.

- Sore mouth.

- Dry, itchy or sore skin.

Radiotherapy

- Nausea.

- Fatigue.

- Sore skin.

- Skin burns.

- Internal discomfort and pain, e.g. mouth, bladder, rectum or whatever part is being treated.

- Hair loss.

- Risk of lymphoedema.

Surgery

- Scarring.

- Tightness.

- Pain and swelling.

- Loss of range of motion.

- Loss of muscle tone or muscle mass.

- Wound.

- Infection.

- Trauma.

- Possible loss of an organ or body part.

- Risk of lymphoedema.

Tumour or lump

- May be 'felt'.

- May be impacting on other organ, tissues or joints.

- Nerve impact may cause pain, loss of sensation or paralysis.

Stoma

- Ileostomy and colostomy: Openings of the large bowel onto the surface of abdomen. The person wears a bag over the opening to collect the bowel contents that would normally be passed. They may be temporary or permanent.

- Tracheostomy: An opening created at the front of the neck so a tube can be inserted into the windpipe (trachea) to help the person breathe.

- 'PEG' or 'PEJ' (percutaneous endoscopic gastrostomy/ jejunostomy): For those with long-term problems with eating and swallowing, such as cancer of the head and neck or oesophagus. It is inserted into the stomach or jejunum through an opening made on the outside of the abdomen. Liquid nutrition is delivered through the tube.

Breathing problems

- Coughing or choking sensations due to the cancer or as a side effect of treatments particularly to the neck or throat.

- Breathlessness: May be due to lack of lung capacity, low blood oxygen or anxiety.

- Tracheostomy – see above.

Cancer in the bones

- Bones may be brittle or fragile.

- Bone metastases.

- Osteoporosis.

- Tumour may be compressing nerves, which may cause numbness, pins and needles, loss of sensation or paralysis.

- Pain and stiffness.

- Loss of range of motion.

Intravenous (IV) access

- 'Hickman' line: A type of 'central line', giving direct access to a large vein. A tube is inserted underneath the chest wall skin and into the large vein draining into the heart. Part of the Hickman line tube remains outside of the skin to give medications or to take blood samples. It usually stays in place for several months or longer.

- 'PICC' line (peripherally inserted central catheter): Another type of central line that goes into a vein in the arm and runs up the vein inside the arm to a large vein in the chest. It can be left in for several months.

- 'Port': A catheter (tube) with a small reservoir (port) attached to it, sometimes called implantable ports, porta-caths or subcutaneous ports. It can remain in place for several months.

- 'Cannula': A short, thin tube that is put into a vein in the crook of the arm or the back of the hand for treatment. It is usually removed before going home. If the person does not have a central line fitted, they will need to be cannulated each time they receive treatment.

In all cases, the area may be sensitive. IV lines are at risk of infection, blockage or blood clots.

Infection

- Infections due to treatments or IV lines.

- Virus, cold, etc.

- Risk to other patients and taxing to the body.

Co-morbidity
Co-morbidity means that someone has more than one presenting medical condition. It is not uncommon that people who are diagnosed with cancer also have a diagnosis of heart disease, diabetes or some other health condition.

Peripheral neuropathy

- Possible side effect of chemotherapy.

- Loss of sensation, numbness or tingling in extremities, especially the hands and feet.

Pain relief

- Effect of opiate drugs, e.g. constipation, sleepiness, confusion, sometimes hallucination.

- Awareness of pain might be dulled.

Oedema and lymphoedema

- Lymphoedema is a possible complication of lymph node removal.

- Oedema is fluid retention often related to surgery or other treatment.

- Do not rule out the risk of DVT (see below) with swelling that has an unknown cause.

Deep vein thrombosis (DVT) and blood clots

- Possible complication of chemotherapy or IV lines.

- A DVT is characterized by unexplained pain in the leg that does not go away, swelling and heat.

- IF CONCERNED, SEEK MEDICAL ADVICE.

Blood pressure

- Can fluctuate significantly with treatments – adapt as appropriate.

Health questionnaire

Taking a health questionnaire is good practice, especially when working with people who have cancer or any other health condition. The first thing to bear in mind is that a person with cancer may also have other health conditions (what is described in medicine as 'co-morbidity'), so it's important not just to ask questions about their cancer. It is quite common for people experiencing cancer to also have cardiovascular conditions or diabetes. This is partly because of age (the risk for all of these things goes up with age) and partly because the risk factors for these conditions are similar.

Although you may already use a basic health questionnaire for your students or clients, here is a list of conditions you should ask about:

- Heart or circulatory conditions.

- High or low blood pressure.

- Diabetes.

- Glaucoma or detached retina (or risk of).

- Epilepsy.

- Asthma or respiratory problems.

- Allergies.

- Back or neck problems, sciatica.

- Joint or bone problems, e.g. arthritis, osteoporosis, brittle bones.

- Mental health problems.

- Pregnancy.

- Medications. If you don't recognize the names, that's okay, but you do need to know what they're taking them for. (This may also alert you to any health issues they haven't told you about.)

Next, ask questions about their cancer:

- What is their diagnosis?

- Details, especially if it's a cancer you are unfamiliar with. Where is the cancer? Or if they have/had something like breast or lung cancer, which side?

- When were they diagnosed?

- What treatments did they have/are they having?

- Are they on any medication?

- Did they have surgery? When?

- Are their surgical wounds healed?

- What side effects are they experiencing?

  - Pain

  - Nausea

  - Diarrhoea

- Fatigue

- Anaemia/low blood counts

- Dizziness, etc.

And these are things to ask every time you see them:

- How are they feeling today?

- Has anything changed since you last saw them?

- How is their blood pressure today?

- How did they feel after the last session?

At the beginning of your first session with the person you will need to allow time to do the health questionnaire. If they are coming along to a general class, you can perhaps email it to them in advance and ask them to fill it out and bring it with them. You could also do it over the phone. Remember that they will probably also need to ask for their doctor's okay to practise yoga if they are still going through treatment or are affected by their condition. This is best practice for any condition that affects someone's physical ability.

Set and setting

▨ QUESTION FOR REFLECTION

Reflect on what you feel would help and what would hinder you in creating an appropriate space to work with someone with a cancer, or their loved ones.

In talking about creating an appropriate environment, the focus can be on the physical aspects of the space that you are working in, and this can, of course, be very important. The space itself, the lighting, the sounds, smells, heating, equipment and possible distractions all play a part in creating a space that is comfortable, welcoming and accessible. There are many practicalities, and as each person has unique needs, you cannot always anticipate what might be required, but concentrating on the basics is a good start.

If you are working in your own space, obviously this is much easier to achieve, but you may be required to meet people in their own homes, in hospital or hospice settings, or in community settings, where your control over the environment is limited. These settings are not always as restful as you might like them to be.

In a typical hospital setting it is actually quite normal for healthcare professionals to interrupt other professionals' sessions with patients, often without even knocking on the door. This is not best practice, but the pressures of time and urgency mean that it does often happen in reality. This can unintentionally undermine the patient's right to choose how, when and where they receive treatment and to a level of privacy that they would be afforded elsewhere. But it happens.

For example, I used to teach a small group of people who attended a yoga class for palliative care. During the hospice refurbishment we were using the rehab gym, temporarily borrowed from the hospital physiotherapy team. It was booked out each week at the same time.

The gym itself was stark and sterile, with a hard floor, uncomfortable chairs and strip lighting. I had to improvise, making the best use of natural daylight, mats borrowed from the gym store to place underfoot, and gentle music playing on my mobile phone. Every week, without fail, one or more members of the physio team would come in – unannounced and unapologetic – to collect a piece of equipment. Often they would do so right in the middle of relaxtion!

I have, in the past, in a boldly and strangely self-righteous fashion, tried to use the opportunity to explain that yoga involves relaxation and that it is not appropriate to interrupt, especially not without asking. Perhaps understandably this has not always been met with the level of understanding that I would have liked. I have clearly trodden on professional toes. This has been an important learning experience for me in acknowledging the need to adapt to the methods and practices of the place that I am working in. So nowadays I gauge whether it is going to be useful, practical and diplomatic before I decide whether to say anything. If it isn't going to change anything, it is better to find a way to adapt.

It is not always possible – even with a promising room, lighting, smells, sounds and quiet – to create the ideal physical space. We can only do our best, and in being prepared to offer our presence to the person with cancer, we, the teachers, are offering a space of ease, compassion and unconditional love. Ultimately, the most important adjustment that teachers can make to the environment is in themselves.

Space and equipment

■ QUESTIONS FOR REFLECTION

Why do you think it is important to create a comfortable environment for people who are living with cancer to practise yoga? What aspects of the space and equipment would be essential for you, and what do you think you could manage or get around?

As a minimum, the space you use should be:

- Clean and hygienic: Avoiding infection is really important, especially for people whose immune system may be compromised. This means that everything you use, e.g. props, needs to be clean/cleanable.

- Accessible for people who are less mobile: If your usual yoga space is up three flights of stairs and there is no lift, you might need to find an alternative venue!

- A comfortable temperature, with the ability to adjust the heat up or down.

- Well ventilated: Ideally windows that open. Rooms with no windows can feel stuffy and claustrophobic. Consider smells – cooking smells can trigger nausea.

- With easy access to a toilet: Cancer treatments can cause diarrhoea, nausea, bladder and bowel issues.

In addition, these aspects are also good to have but might be worked around if the space is otherwise okay:

- Well-lit with natural light and/or gentle electric lighting.

- Blinds or curtains that can be drawn over windows if there is strong sunlight.

- Tastefully decorated and uncluttered.

- Access to good, clean yoga equipment.

- Free of interruptions.

- Away from noisy areas.

If you are working in your own space, meeting these requirements is probably much easier than in a rented space. You may also meet people in their own homes where you might end up working in tiny spaces cluttered with hamster cages or laundry. You may be disturbed by the sounds of children, dogs, partners, doorbells, phones and all of the other usual interruptions of domestic life.

In hospital, hospice or community settings, you may need to work in a clinical area, interrupted by healthcare practitioners and people coming in to offer tea, the sound of medical equipment, noisy vacuum cleaners and the sound of other patients, and you may not have access to the ideal equipment.

There will be scenarios where you have to improvise, carry equipment with you, and take all the other trappings to turn a space into a temporary relaxing space. Wherever I go, I carry the following portable 'yogi kit' with me:

- Candle. I use a battery-operated LED candle where naked flames are not appropriate.

- An aromatherapy space-clearing spray to prepare the space before people arrive. Australian Bush Flower Clearing Spray is one of my favourites that you can buy from shops like Neal's Yard. But you can find other ready-made sprays in health food and 'new age' shops and even some pharmacies. If you are qualified in the use of aromatherapy oils, you may wish to blend your own. Avoid anything with artificial perfumes or chemicals, and always be mindful of allergies and sensitivity to smells.

- A portable Bluetooth speaker that connects with a phone

to play relaxing music, or even just a phone that has a good enough speaker for a small space.

▨ QUESTIONS FOR REFLECTION

Consider the space you use for your classes at present. How would it be suitable or adaptable, or not? With all equipment consider infection control and hygiene. How do you clean the equipment between use? Soft furnishings are not so easily wiped down. What arrangements would you make for laundry? Would you encourage people to have their own props for hygiene reasons?

Language and metaphor

Words have power: power to hurt and to heal; power to transmit messages of love and compassion; and power to cause insult, injury and pain. In yogic terms, they hold vibration and energy. When I encounter a person living with cancer, I want to promote the energy of healing. Of living, rather than surviving. Of healing, rather than fighting. Of personhood, rather than patient-hood. This way of speaking is often called 'person first' language. It acknowledges that a person is NOT their condition but rather a person living with a condition.

There is some debate about the types of words and especially the metaphors that we use to describe the experience of cancer. Metaphors are words and phrases or stories that we invent to describe situations, events and people that are not actually about those things. The most common ones we have all encountered – because they are so ubiquitous – are those that equate cancer to a battle, war or fighting. Perhaps they are so ubiquitous that you hadn't thought about them as metaphors:

He lost his three-year battle with cancer.
Together we will win the war on cancer.
The best cancer-fighting foods.

Violence imagery and language is the most common, and some people think it's motivational, but for many people experiencing cancer it is quite the opposite. It carries connotations, as battles do, of winning and losing, and with losing, failure. If someone doesn't want to fight but make friends with their cancer, they can face extraordinary pressure from loved ones who think that fighting is the right thing to do. Additionally, the energy of fighting causes the same fight, flight, freeze or fold sympathetic nervous system response in the body that we are trying to minimize and help by practising yoga. Minimizing stress and its effects on the body is a major factor in recovery, and if the person is not going to survive, of helping them to live with a better sense of peace and harmony while they are alive.

In her 2014 article for *The Guardian*, 'Having cancer is not a fight or a battle',[6] Dr Kate Granger – who died from cancer in 2016 – said, 'I refuse to believe my death will be because I didn't battle hard enough.'

If something feels empowering to a person, then I do not challenge. However, I don't use the language myself, and I encourage my students to avoid fighting language and use person first language in relation to cancer too. This models the principle that we are working first with the person, and not just their cancer. I tend to use the terms 'living with cancer' and 'person experiencing cancer'. I choose not to use the words 'cancer survivor', 'survivorship', 'battle' or 'fight' in relation to cancer. The metaphors we choose can affect how we relate to and how we approach our illness.

EXERCISE

You may be interested in reading the article 'May I take your metaphor? – how we talk about cancer'[7] from Cancer Research UK about using battle-type language and other metaphors around cancer. The video included in the article, with Professor Elena Semino, explains some of the research around both the motivations for fundraisers and the disempowerment felt by individuals.

CHAPTER TWO

Satya

It is easier
to tell the truth. That way
everything is clear.

The second Yama is Satya, which, in its most basic translation, means honesty or truthfulness. In a therapeutic context, honesty and transparency about who we are, and what we are able to offer, are vital for trust. When people are diagnosed with cancer, they often research and seek out complementary and alternative treatments that they have heard might be of benefit, and yoga is one of them.

People seek out complementary therapies like yoga because they have hope that it will help them feel better, cope with treatments better, and survive longer. Sometimes people seek out alternative treatments because they are hoping for a cure. And there are any number of unscrupulous practitioners who are ready to take their money. This is dishonest and unethical.

Yoga is not a cure for cancer, but it does have many benefits. The important thing is that we communicate honestly about what the benefits are, from an evidence-based perspective.

In this chapter we look at the benefits of Yoga for Cancer and some of the scientific evidence base, and then at some of the myths around cancer and its treatment.

The benefits of Yoga for Cancer
Complementary therapy

Yoga can be hugely helpful in enabling people to cope with the side effects of their treatments. It can also be considered a complementary therapy. We use the term 'complementary' to describe supportive therapies such as massage, Reiki, reflexology and yoga because these treatments are considered by the medical profession to be effective and safe only alongside, or complementary to, conventional treatments.

Reading though the list of side effects in the previous chapter, you can see how yoga might be very beneficial to people who are going through treatment for cancer, not only in relieving some of the physical side effects of treatment, but also in helping them to cope with the emotional, spiritual and psychological effects of a cancer diagnosis and treatment.

Thankfully, yoga is generally accepted and advocated as a safe complementary practice by oncology professionals and cancer charities. And now that we have a growing body of reliable clinical evidence, offering yoga to people living with cancer is getting much easier. Most people still see yoga as a gentle way to exercise the body, but much of the emerging evidence is showing (as if we needed proof) that there is more to yoga than just stretching! We still have a few hills to climb, but we're getting there.

■ **QUESTIONS FOR REFLECTION**

What is the difference between a complementary therapy and an alternative therapy? Why do you think yoga is considered to be a complementary therapy?

The science

We are now seeing a good body of evidence-based material emerging that supports what yogis have known for a very long time. And that is that this yoga stuff seems to work!

A lot of the existing evidence about yoga and cancer relates to self-reported 'quality of life' measures such as social function, happiness and so on, and this is quite conclusive. But science is very much focused on more objective measurements, and studies are also beginning to show that yoga regulates levels of the stress-regulating steroid hormone cortisol in the bodies of people with cancer. (For more on cortisol, see below.) There is good solid evidence demonstrating stress reduction through yoga in the general population, and now studies are showing that yoga also has a stress-reducing effect specifically in people going through cancer treatment – more to add to the evidence base.

A ground-breaking study led by the Centre for Integrative Studies at the MD Anderson Cancer Center in Texas, USA was published in the *Journal of Clinical Oncology* in 2014. It stated that yoga 'improved quality of life and physiological changes associated with radiotherapy treatment' and – this is the important bit – that the benefits offered by yoga went 'beyond [those] of simple stretching exercises, and these benefits appear to have long-term durability'.[8]

Cortisol

The study used cortisol as a quantitative measure. Cortisol is a steroid hormone that has an important role in helping the body respond to stress; hence it is often referred to as a 'stress hormone'. Cortisol also regulates a wide range of processes throughout the body, including metabolism and the immune response. Cortisol peaks in the morning and, in a typical circadian rhythm, tapers off steeply through the day. In people who are chronically stressed, this tapering pattern flattens out, meaning that cortisol in the bloodstream remains relatively high. Yoga seems to have a significant impact on this dysfunctional pattern: people who practise yoga tend to have a steeper decline in their cortisol levels throughout the day.

Stress and the mind–body connection

There is a current field of research called psychoneuroimmunology (PNI). It describes the pathways and connection between the mind and the immune system – via the nervous system. You may also encounter it as psychoneuroendocrinoimmunology (PNEI), correctly emphasizing the role of the endocrine functions in the holistic picture. Basically, science is catching up with what has been widely understood in traditional medicine modalities for some time, and that is that you cannot separate the mind from the body when looking at cancer, or at any other disease. A 2014 article in *Brain, Behavior, and Immunity*[9] cites some significant research in this area.

One of the most well known proponents of this field of study is Dr Gabor Maté who says in his book, *When the Body Says No*,[10] that our emotions and our hormonal, immune and nervous systems are interconnected. Therefore stress, especially chronic stress, intrinsically and inevitably has an effect on all of the body's systems. The book is well worth a read for an accessible and compelling approach to this fascinating area of study.

More clinical evidence

This section contains various links to published clinical research. Unless you are a geek like me, you might not wish to read the entire published articles. You can generally get the information you need from the abstract and/or conclusion at the beginning of each article, and these are often published even if the full article requires payment.

Agarwal and Maroko-Afek (2018) 'Yoga into cancer care: A review of the evidence-based research':[11] This review article presents the published clinical research on the use of yoga with people living with cancer, with most of the studies cited showing yoga improved the physical and psychological symptoms, quality of life and markers of immunity of the patients.

Kiecolt-Glaser *et al.* (2014) 'Yoga's impact on inflammation, mood, and fatigue in breast cancer survivors: A randomized controlled trial', Conclusions:[12] Chronic inflammation may fuel declines in physical function leading to frailty and disability. If yoga dampens or limits both fatigue and inflammation, then regular practice could have substantial health benefits.

Bower *et al.* (2014) 'Yoga reduces inflammatory signaling in fatigued breast cancer survivors', Conclusions:[13] A 12-week restorative Iyengar Yoga intervention reduced inflammation-related gene expression in breast cancer survivors with persistent fatigue. These findings suggest that a targeted yoga programme may have beneficial effects on inflammatory activity in this patient population, with potential relevance for behavioural and physical health

If you would like to do your own searches on published evidence, research or reviews, then you can use a paper search engine such as Google Scholar or PubMed[14] and search for yoga + cancer.

Myth busting

If you are a yoga teacher, the chances are that you are also familiar with, or indeed fully immersed in the world of, alternative therapies. I am additionally trained as a practitioner in massage, Reiki and Bach Flower Remedies (to name just a few of my flurry of certificates), and I very much enjoy using incense, candles and crystals. But (there was inevitably a 'but') I am extremely wary of anything alternative that claims to 'cure' cancer, and of any pseudo-scientific ideas about what causes cancer.

So here, in no particular order, is my myth-busting list of the three most common ideas you will encounter. In all cases, I have included the truth that lurks in all the ideas, as all myths start somewhere.

A loving note before we start. It is possible that you hold some of these ideas. My encouragement is to gently notice your reaction and be kind to it. I am not insisting that you let go of any beliefs that you have; however, it is important, if you are going to be working with people with cancer, that you don't offer any ideas that are contrary to medical opinion or that encourage people to try alternative approaches. Remember – someone living with a cancer diagnosis is extremely vulnerable, and may well take your advice to heart. Support them in their own choices.

Myth #1: Sugar 'feeds' cancer

This is an extremely popular and pervasive idea, because it *sounds* true. And on one basic biological level, it is true. It is true in that all cells in the body require sugar (in the form of glucose) as an energy supply. Because cancer cells grow faster than normal cells, they have a higher demand for glucose.

What isn't true is that eating sugar or sugary foods directly feeds cancer (or any other cell). This isn't how the biology works; it is way more complex. All of the food we eat is broken down into various nutrients and the glucose is used as an energy supply. Cancer cells, like all other cells, require a host of nutrients to grow and multiply.

Consuming too many calories will invariably be stored in the body as fat, and being overweight is a risk factor for many cancers. Additionally, people who eat a lot of sugary foods are less likely to eat fruit and vegetables, which is another risk factor.

Take away: Do not tell anyone to cut out sugar from their diet. When they are having treatment, sugary foods may be the only thing they can stomach, which is supplying them with much needed calories.

Myth #2: Cancer is 'acidic' and an 'alkaline' diet can cure it

You can hear me uttering a big sigh when I hear this theory. It works on the idea that cancer does not thrive in an overly alkaline environment. This bit is true, but then neither can any of our normal cells. What is profoundly unscientific, however, is the idea that what we eat can directly alter the body's pH.[15] As a result of homeostasis, the pH level of our blood remains slightly alkaline, because of a biological process that is very tightly managed by the kidneys. What we eat has no effect on this process, and any excess alkalinity or acidity is excreted in urine. Because the so-called 'alkaline' foods are plants, then it is inevitably a healthier diet that contains more fruit and vegetables. But it has no measurable impact on blood alkalinity.

Take away: More fruit and vegetables is good, and to be encouraged, but it does nothing to change our pH.

Myth #3: Cannabis oil cures cancer

CBD (cannabidiol) oil is really popular as a supplement, and many people use it for its pain relieving and anti-inflammatory properties. I use it. However, there is no evidence that it prevents or cures cancer or kills cancer cells. What is true is that – in the laboratory environment – certain cannabis compounds (cannabinoids) do kill cancer cells (and healthy cells), stop cells dividing, and stop cells creating a blood supply. However, the chemicals have also been found to damage important blood vessels.

Other studies have very mixed results. Some show that cannabis can reduce cancer risk and others have shown that it can actually increase cancer risk. The use of CBD oil may also interfere with some medicines, including chemotherapy. Additionally, because CBD oil and other cannabis products are unregulated, there is no way of tightly managing the dose, or of ensuring the medical purity of the product.

Take away: CBD is a potent medicine and has its uses in many conditions. However, even if you personally swear by it, do not advocate the use of CBD oil for someone going through cancer treatment. If they tell you they are taking it, or thinking of taking it, encourage them to talk to their medical team about whether it is appropriate for them.

EXERCISE

Research some other common cancer 'myths' on the internet and look at the scientific evidence relating to each. Reflect on how you will communicate with someone who advocates some of these beliefs in relation to their own treatment.

CHAPTER THREE

Asteya

I find true wealth in
not stealing anyone's time,
energy or trust.

The topics in this chapter are hung around the idea that Asteya – or non-stealing – goes further than the principle of simply not taking a material object that does not belong to us. Hopefully, that one goes without saying!

Stealing might also refer to the misuse of someone's time, trust, energy or vulnerability. This could apply to overreaching or mis-selling our abilities and qualifications, or to breaching someone's confidentiality and right to consent, or to the use of someone else's experience of suffering to satisfy a personal need to help.

Be prepared in this chapter for a bumpy, but ultimately fruitful, journey of examining your own practice and motivations.

Scope of practice

We have all had students who will come up to us at the end of a class and ask for advice. Over the years I have been asked for advice on topics ranging from ankle injuries to detox diets to relationships! Sound familiar? And how tempting it is to try to help when someone asks for it.

I still remember a phrase that I was encouraged to repeat during my massage training. It served as a mantra to remind us of our scope of practice:

We are not doctors. We do not treat. We do not diagnose!

You may, of course, BE a doctor, in which case, you will know better than I do about where the scope of your practice begins and where it ends. A fellow yoga teacher who is also a practising GP does not dispense medical advice in the yoga room. Her answer to any student with a medical question is for them to go and speak to their own GP! And this should be the answer that any non-medical person should give to a medical question: 'I don't know. I encourage you to seek medical advice.'

Whilst I acknowledge that many yoga teachers are additionally qualified in many different disciplines such as massage, acupuncture, psychotherapy or nutrition, it is important that unless you are properly qualified, *you do not*:

- Treat injuries – although you can, of course, assist in modifying the yoga practice for injuries, and you can administer first aid if an injury occurs in class.

- Give advice about diet and nutrition, including supplements. You can talk about the benefits of, for example, a vegetarian diet, without preaching.

- Offer opinions about the efficacy – or otherwise – of conventional treatments.

- Offer massage.

- Recommend the use of, or administer products like, essential oils, herbal remedies or flower tinctures for self-treatment.

- Offer counselling for psychological or emotional issues. You can, of course, offer a space to listen and be present.

- Make any unsubstantiated medical claims about the practice of yoga – although you can talk about the established benefits and the scientific evidence relating to yoga and cancer.

The reasons

- It should be clear – to the student, to you and to everyone else – what your role is in the yoga room. This avoids any overstepping of boundaries.

- It is misleading to allow people to believe that you are qualified to offer advice or treatments that you are not qualified to give.

- We do not need any more reasons to undermine the professionalism of yoga teaching!

- In some cases, it is illegal to make certain health claims, e.g. about supplements.

- You will not be insured for offering these things, so in the (hopefully unlikely) event that someone makes a claim against you, you may find yourself without financial or legal cover.

The wounded healer

You may have come across the idea and concept of the 'wounded healer'. It has its origins in Greek Mythology, although it was introduced as a psychoanalytical concept by the psychologist Carl Jung, who also explored the idea of archetypes. Jung's idea is that the therapist (counsellor, psychotherapist, healer, yoga teacher?) is compelled to help people because of their own emotional and psychological wounds.

This does not mean that if you carry wounds – and we all do – you should not be doing your job. The archetype also suggests that as well as being drawn to healing because of a person's own need for healing, their own wounds can be a significant strength in helping others. I include it here because these motivations can easily move from a strength to a burden. If you are aware that your own traumas, wounds and need for healing form at least part of your own experience, and indeed a part of your desire to help others, it helps you to maintain a visible and healthy awareness of it.

Another thing to be aware of is how the healer impulse can have its shadow side. This might include impulses like trying to fix or 'rescue' people, experiencing a 'need to be needed', helping people without their request (that is, whether they want to be helped or not), feeling like a hero or a martyr, doing so much that you risk burnout, giving people unsolicited advice, etc.

To maintain a healthy relationship with your ' healer':

- Look at, and be honest about, what you are doing and why. What are your motivations for helping? Is it your job to be helping in that way?

- Learn to hold your own boundaries with compassion. Know where you end and the other person begins. Where are the boundaries blurry?

- Accept the limits of your expertise. Accept not knowing. Are you taking on roles outside of your scope of practice?

- Practise being present when the need to 'do' something comes up. Is it your stuff? Or does something actually need to happen to help the other person be more comfortable?

- Know when it is appropriate to refer to other professionals, defer to family members or, perhaps most importantly, allow the person to be in full agency around their choices.

- Engage in regular professional supervision (see more on this in Chapter Nine).

The wounded healer is one aspect of the healer archetype, one of 12 archetypes suggested by Jung as descriptors of the mythical and universal characteristics that reside in the collective unconscious, that we all embody to some degree or another. You might want to do some further reading, and there are plenty of resources on the internet. If you have a desire to go deeper into the thoughts of Jung, The Society of Analytical Psychology[16] has some excellent free re-sources. You may also be interested in Henri Nouwen's book, *The Wounded Healer.*[17]

■ **QUESTIONS FOR REFLECTION**

Where might your own experience be influencing your desire to help people living with cancer? How might that be a strength? Where might your desire to help fall into 'shadow'?

Confidentiality

When you are working with people with medical conditions like cancer, you are generally party to their personal and medical history. They may also share with you some deep feelings or intimate physical details. All of this is between you and the person. Nobody else. Not your partner, not your fellow teachers.

There are some circumstances in which it may be acceptable to share some details. For example, if you work in a clinical setting, where other practitioners have access to the patient and their medical notes, then it might be considered appropriate to share certain information. You might also share some information with the person you have nominated as your supervisor or mentor, for the purposes of support, but otherwise, what you are told in confidence remains that way, unless the person gives you express permission to share it. If someone shares something about themselves that may be revealed in class, then always ask what they want others to know. They may not be ready to, or want to share it publicly. And it can be so easy to accidentally blurt something out.

The law

The law requires that 'Information given in confidence must not be disclosed without consent unless there is a justifiable reason, e.g. a requirement of law or there is an overriding public interest to do so.'[18] Which begs the question of course – what are justifiable reasons?

This may sometimes be less clear cut than others, BUT if you believe that a person, or someone in their care, is at serious risk of harm, or if a serious crime has been committed, then those are reasons someone might choose to disclose to someone in authority. If the police request to see someone's notes because a crime has been committed, that may be another reason.

If you are working on behalf of an organization, they should have their own protocols around confidentiality, safeguarding and disclosure that you should adhere to. But ultimately, you are responsible for the safekeeping of any information that you hold on your clients.

Notes, records or personal information that you hold about a person should be stored and handled in strict accordance with the General Data Protection Regulation (GDPR).[19]

Medical consent

It is advisable that your students who are living with a diagnosis of cancer obtain permission from their consultant, specialist nurse or their GP to practise yoga, especially if they have a complex condition that could be affected by the practice. If someone has recovered from their medical treatment and is no longer experiencing any strong effects, either of the condition or its treatment (for example, it has been a few years since they had treatment), then it might be okay to accept them into a class without having their doctor's go-ahead. In fact, the doctor would probably find the question rather strange.

As a general rule of thumb, if someone is having treatment, or they are still living with their cancer as a long-term or recurring illness, get them to ask their doctor if it is okay. You don't need to get this in writing from the doctor – in truth, you might be waiting a long time! They can simply ask at a routine or telephone appointment and get their doctor to say it is okay. Then they can sign your consent form to state that this is the case. Generally, people who approach me because they have read that yoga is something that might help them have usually asked their consultant about it already.

Although many doctors are now aware what yoga is, there are still many misconceptions about it, so you may wish to create a handout describing a basic yoga practice, and how it is adapted for someone living with cancer, so that the doctor knows what is involved.

Sensitivity

You will come face to face with the physical manifestations of the person's illness or treatment, some of which you may find difficult to witness or even find physically repellent. Dealing with these things with gentle sensitivity is really important, as the person will probably already be feeling rather self-conscious or even embarrassed. When you have prepared for something in your imagination, it is always easier to deal with in reality.

◼ QUESTIONS FOR REFLECTION

Consider how you might need to make accommodations or manage the following sensitivities in your class. Think about how you might need to make adjustments within yourself too!

- A person with a colostomy bag[20] (that may need to be emptied).

- A person whose condition or treatment causes them to suffer from nosebleeds.

- A person whose treatment causes them to have a strong and unpleasant body odour.

- A person who may have a sudden urge to vomit.

Do you have any feelings of revulsion around other bodily functions that you may need to address?

CHAPTER FOUR

Brahmacharya

Clear boundaries and
resilient energy.
My spirit is strong.

Brahmacharya is a much misunderstood and difficult concept for most Western practitioners of yoga to get their heads around, mostly because it is interpreted in many paths as celibacy, and this is not a popular idea. In literal terms it means conduct that is consistent with, or on the path of, Brahman. Brahman is the Universal Consciousness or Ultimate Reality that some people equate with God. Being on the path of Brahman suggests conduct that is in alignment with our concept of the Universe, the Divine, or our own highest nature.

Traditionally, this refers to various forms of self-restraint that are conducive to the practices of yoga and to the spiritual paths of Buddhism, Hinduism and Jainism. As modern practitioners of yoga we might interpret it as the *right use of energy*. And so, this chapter focuses largely on the exploration of boundaries – physical, emotional, professional and energetic.

Boundaries

QUESTION FOR REFLECTION

Before you read further, think about what is meant by boundaries. You might want to think about this question from the point of view of personal boundaries and professional boundaries, and what this means in relation to working with people with cancer. Capture your thoughts.

Personal boundaries might be thought of as the ways in which a person identifies or ensures safety for themselves and others in terms of how they behave towards others, and how they accept or limit the ways in which others behave towards them.

Have a think about how you manage your own personal boundaries. You may wish to reflect on, and then make notes about, the following questions. In each case, think also about how you feel, and how you might develop a stronger (or less rigid) boundary:

- In what circumstances do I find it difficult to say no?

- How do I share personal information about myself?

- How do I react when others share opinions that I strongly disagree with?

Professional boundaries

The British Association for Counselling and Psychotherapy (BACP)[21] defines boundaries as follows:

> The limits in relationships between practitioners and their clients that, if crossed, could cause harm to the client or contravene professional standards and ethics.

The BACP then goes on to define in some detail where those boundaries should lie within the framework of a strict code of ethics. Appropriate boundaries are very much dependent on context. We have different boundaries for personal relationships than for professional relationships. And the nature of the professional relationship will determine what is appropriate too.

Yoga intimately deals with the whole person, and is essentially therapeutic in its practice. Even if that is not the focus of a yoga class, people will come to class hoping to feel better physically, emotionally and psychologically. This puts the yoga teacher in a position of trust, and, as the one leading the class, in a relative position of power to the student. When people come to yoga with a diagnosis of cancer, and especially if they have an expectation that the yoga will help them in some way, then the relationship is a therapeutic one. An understanding of therapeutic professional boundaries is, therefore, a necessity.

This is a contentious issue when there is a 'blurring' of boundaries, when the boundary between professional and personal relationship becomes less clear. This does not mean it is wrong to blur the boundaries sometimes, but it does require the person in the position of relative power to have really good discrimination and to know, very clearly, and for very good reasons, where the ultimate edges of those boundaries lie, and if needs be, to hold those boundaries on behalf of the student who may not be so clear.

▓ QUESTION FOR REFLECTION

Reflect on the following scenario, and note your thoughts around the boundaries of the following situation:

> Clare runs a weekly yoga class at a local cancer centre on a Monday morning. There is a relatively new student, Tony, who has just been diagnosed with colon cancer, and who seems to need a lot of support. He approaches Clare at the end of the class to ask for some advice about his practice, and then asks her if she would like to go for a coffee. She is not sure if he is attracted to her, as he is generally very open and friendly with everyone.

Touch

Touch is a powerful, and necessary, aspect of human existence. All human beings need touch, and indeed it is essential to our well-being. Conscious, consensual touch can be nurturing, healing and deeply caring. Navigating the boundaries of appropriate touch can be tricky in the student–teacher relationship, and especially in the case of people going through cancer treatment, when the student is additionally vulnerable. During cancer treatment, the regular kind of touch that people receive is clinical, it is often detached, and it can be invasive, involving needles, injections and lots of discomfort and pain, so touch offered in the spirit of comfort and kindness is often very gratefully received. However, for the same reasons, touch – which may feel like more 'being done to' – may not be desired at all. We can be sensitive around offering touch by seeking consent and establishing boundaries and being aware of trauma sensitivity.

Until very recently, it has been the habit in many yoga classes, particularly the more dynamic styles, to adjust students, and to do so without seeking any form of explicit consent. If your teacher training was a while ago, it maybe wasn't even raised as an issue. Certainly, when I trained, it was customary to walk around the class and give adjustments to everyone, without asking. It was just expected that this would happen. This is what is now referred to as *implied consent*, meaning that the student was considered to be giving their consent to be adjusted by being in the class in the first place. Some teachers still operate on this basis.

However, as yoga teachers are becoming (hopefully) more trauma sensitive and more aware of consent issues all round, it is becoming more and more common to at least ask the person's permission to touch them before you offer an adjustment or any other kind of touch. I no longer physically adjust my students' postures, and I myself generally find it invasive to be adjusted. If I touch, it is gentle, guiding and encouraging. This is partly because I work with people living with cancer, and adjusting people usually isn't appropriate, but my practice has also evolved to consider this best practice all round. I do recognize, however, that some students enjoy hands-on adjustments and look forward to them. And, of course, as we establish ongoing trusting relationships with our students, and learn how they tick, the dynamic of consent and touch becomes easier to navigate. However, the key to offering any kind of touch is always consent.

How, then, do you establish consent? Can you assume that the absence of a no, or saying nothing, constitutes a yes? Can you rely on people telling you that they don't want to be touched? The trauma-sensitive approach is that consent to touch should be opt in and not opt out – meaning, a person should say a definite YES to being touched. There are many complex reasons for this, but at the most basic level, speaking up is difficult for some people in a group setting, so if you say something like, 'If you don't want to be touched, please let me know', this doesn't help the person who would rather just put up with the unwanted touch than draw attention to themselves. Additionally, someone who has been going through lots of medical interventions may have a reduced sense of personal agency and may not have a particular handle on whether they want to be touched or not. This calls for great sensitivity.

Some teachers now use cards, chips or counters that are double-sided which a student can flip over at any time during the class to say, silently, to the teacher whether they are happy with being touched or not. Because it can be really hard to say no for some people, any way of communicating this non-verbally is a very useful tool of empowerment. You can buy commercially produced ones, or I use a double-sided coaster that I bought really cheaply. It has a red side and a green side (red for no, green for yes). People can flip it at any time during the practice. You could even make your own. It just needs to be something you can see and interpret easily.

However, even if you have a *green for go* consent, it is still best practice to ask first. It is as easy as saying something like 'Is it okay if I put my hands on your shoulders/lower back/feet?' If the person says yes, but doesn't seem sure, I ask again; if they still seem unsure, I take it as a no. Some teachers include other visible ways of gaining consent. One teacher I know asks his students to 'wiggle their toes' if they would like to receive a gentle neck and shoulder adjustment in Savasana. No wiggly toes, no adjustment! Note: He still always asks again before he puts his hands on them.

Saying no

Another question to ask is, do your students know it is okay to say no to you? It might seem obvious, but saying no, especially to a teacher – the person in the position of power in the dynamic – is difficult for a lot of people. There is a cultural edge to this, where politeness may often be valued above personal agency. The classic school model of teaching has carried its way into the yoga room and yoga teachers – sometimes even called 'instructors' – carry a lot of power and trust. Think about it – we are in a position to ask a group of grown adults to do things with their bodies that, sometimes even against their own instincts, they will usually try to do.

It is worth letting your students know from the outset that it is okay for them to say no to you. When it comes to touch, you might set this expectation up by saying something like, 'I may offer hands-on assistance in this class. I will always ask if you want to be touched. If you don't want to be touched, it is 100 per cent okay for you to say no to me. I will never be offended by you making a choice that is right for you or your body. If you don't feel like speaking, just shake your head. And if you don't say yes, I will take it as a no.'

Touch can be a wonderful thing. And a calming, guiding, loving hand from a trusted teacher can be a healing and nurturing gift. But for some, being touched can feel invasive. And like our moods, this can change from day to day. We can't assume that because someone said yes last week, that they will today.

The answer is consent. Just ask.

Accessibility and inclusion

Understanding inclusion is a way of ensuring that your services – in this case, teaching Yoga for Cancer – are fair and accessible and that nobody is discriminated against because of their colour, physical or mental ability, gender, sexual orientation, values, beliefs, culture or lifestyle.

Those receiving treatment for cancer bring with them all of their other identities – in addition to the difficulties that go along with their cancer diagnosis – which may mean that they are less able to access a yoga class or teacher, or less able to advocate for themselves. There are also particular issues around health inequalities for specific groups who find access to healthcare more difficult, and who have particular experiences of discrimination when accessing healthcare, including cancer services. This is especially the case for people from Black and Minority Ethnic/Black, Indigenous and People of Color (BAME/BIPOC) communities, older people and LGBTQ+ people. Macmillan Cancer Support[22] has some excellent resources that I urge you to read in relation to health inequalities. Their 'No one overlooked' publications give some context to some of the barriers that people face, which are equally relevant to us as yoga teachers.

Equality: What does the law say?

The (UK) Equality Act 2010 lists nine protected characteristics, meaning that it is illegal to discriminate against, or provide less favourable treatment to, a person based on these particular characteristics. This applies to access to services as well as to employment. You can find more detailed outlines on each point from the Equality and Human Rights Commission,[23] which you are encouraged to read. There may be some areas that you are less familiar with, and these might be the ones that you explore in more detail.

- Age.
- Disability.
- Gender reassignment.
- Marriage and civil partnership.
- Pregnancy and maternity.
- Race.
- Religion or belief.
- Sex.
- Sexual orientation.

Diversity acknowledges that differences can be many and varied, and as well as those areas covered by equality law can include:

- Cultural background.
- National origin.
- Region, including accent.
- Gender identity.
- Marital status.
- Political views.
- Ethnicity.
- Socio-economic differences.

- Housing status.

- Family structure.

- Health values.

- Appearance, etc.

Inclusion is about making sure that we make adjustments to how we do things to make our services open and accessible to the range of diversity.

But I treat everyone equally!
I hear this often from yoga teachers, and it is beautiful and laudable. However, there is a difference between treating everyone the same and treating everyone in a way that honours diversity. Diversity acknowledges that far from being the same, we all have diverse needs, and that some aspects of our individuality need to be specifically acknowledged in order to give us fair and equal access to things. And this is at the heart of inclusion. It isn't necessarily enough just to feel inclusive; we have to do things that make our services inclusive. And that means thinking about the potential barriers that there may be.

◼ QUESTIONS FOR REFLECTION

How might you be inadvertently creating barriers to access your services? There may be obvious things, such as your class is upstairs with no lift. But there may be more subtle things that you hadn't thought about.

Think about each of the nine characteristics listed above, and the other areas of diversity, and then consider changes you might make to become more inclusive in your practice. Reflect on the areas of diversity that you might need to know more about, and do some research. Some useful publications are included in the 'Resources to Inform Your Research' section at the end of the book.

This isn't about being 'wrong' in what you are doing, but about opening up the space to include those who might otherwise be excluded, and in turn opening up possibilities for you to have a more inclusive, socially just and rewarding practice!

Looking after yourself

QUESTIONS FOR REFLECTION

How do you practise self-care, and where might you be able to do it better?

One of the most important aspects of working with other people is that you take care of yourself. You are probably already aware of your own tendencies in work and giving. In her book, *Standing at the Edge*,[24] Joan Halifax speaks about the five 'edge states': altruism, empathy, integrity, respect and engagement. She also deals with their shadow sides: pathological altruism, empathic distress, moral suffering, disrespect and burnout.

Chances are that, because you are an engaged and caring person, you have experienced some of these shadow states at some point in your life. You will have come to realize that when you are working for the needs of other people it is vital that you also look after your own needs. This is about making sure that you are compassionate towards your own emotional and physical wellbeing. My teacher Mukunda Stiles said that you cannot afford to be a leaky bucket! In this context, he was talking about leaking energy (Prana) – we must ensure our own 'buckets' of Prana are full, that is, that we are attending to our own needs if we are to be able to fully attend to the needs of others.

How do you fill your bucket?

- Having enough down time. When do you have time to recharge your own Prana 'batteries'?

- Making time for your own practice. If you are teaching yoga and not practising, why is that?

- Have a self-care routine that includes things that you know contribute to your wellbeing – walking, spending time in nature, singing, swimming, art, gardening, massages, whatever works for you.

- If you are working in any way therapeutically with people, seek supervision with another professional who is able to listen to your emotional feedback. (I will talk more about supervision in Chapter Nine.)

Protecting your energy

In yoga, we accept that there is an energetic aspect to the practice. This energy is referred to as Prana, or life force. When you offer a healing space to someone who is going through treatment for cancer, and who is unwell, there is an inevitable draw on this energy that can be very depleting. You do get it back – through rest and, of course, your own yoga practice – but it is better not to allow yourself to be drained in the first place.

Practitioners of all kinds use various 'protection' rituals in preparation for working therapeutically. These vary from very simple and humanistic to religious, esoteric and new age. Truly, they are all helpful because power lies in the intention and focus that you create. I share a few of my favourite methods here, and then list some ideas you might try. The most important thing is that you find something that works for you and that you will remember to do. It is entirely personal to you.

Grounding/centring

One of the easiest and most effective is a grounding or centring technique. This one can be remembered as ABC:

A – Awareness: Be aware of how you are in the present moment. Notice what is present, how you are standing, sitting, holding yourself.

B – Balance: Balance your weight. If you are standing, feel the weight evenly across the soles of your feet. If you are sitting, sit upright with your feet resting on the floor.

Also:

B – Breathing: Be aware of your breath. Breathe easily.

C – Core relaxed: Soft eyes, tongue, chest, belly, and breathing deeply.

C can also mean:

C – Connected: Think of, or picture, a person who makes you feel good.

Shanti Mantra

Shanti, in Sanskrit, means peace. We often chant Shanti after we chant 'Om'. A Shanti Mantra is used to invoke peace and understanding and to create a protected space in which we can learn and practise. This Mantra is often chanted at the beginning of a class or personal practice. This is a phonetic transliteration with the accents on the vowels that are stressed:

Om Saha nāvavatu
saha nau bhunaktu
Saha vīryam karavāvahai
Tejasvi nāvadhītamastu
Mā vidvisāvahai
Om Shānti, Shānti, Shānti.

The Mantra translates as:

Om, May we all be protected
May we all be nourished
May we work together with great energy
May our intellect be sharpened (may our study be effective)
Let there be no animosity amongst us (may we not quarrel)
Om, peace, peace, peace.

You can listen to me chanting this on SoundCloud.[25] Also, if you search 'Om Sahana Vavatu' on the internet, you will find many versions to listen to and enjoy.

'Clearing' your energy, or a space

Many practitioners – and I am one of them – like to clear the energy in the space that they are working in. They might do this before or after receiving a client or class into the space (or both!). There are several ways to do this including using incense smoke, aromatherapy spray, bells, a sound bowl, chanting or clapping. The most important thing is that it feels authentic to you, and that it has meaning for you.

Walk around your space (I usually do this sun-wise/clockwise) with your incense, spray, bells, etc. You can also go around your own 'aura' in the same way. Whatever you do, it is the intention that is important.

Divine Light

A profound and effective way of practising energetic protection is to imagine yourself surrounded by light. The following is a simple technique that I use often:

1. Stand with your feet comfortably apart. Feel your feet connected with the Earth, your weight balanced, your spine long, the crown of your head growing towards the sky.

2. Relax your breath, your face and close your eyes, or take a soft downward gaze.

3. Imagine above the crown of your head a beautiful Divine Light (many people imagine it as white, but your Divine Light may be another colour). Feel that the source of this light is the Divine presence, or whatever source of goodness, light and protection you believe that to be.

4. Then imagine that light pouring down around you and surrounding you completely in light.

5. Breathe easily. You may choose to repeat a mantra or affirmation such as 'I am surrounded and protected by Divine Light.'

6. Practise as long as you feel you need to sustain the feeling

of protection before releasing, taking a deep breath, and moving into your day.

One of my favourite practices is *The Divine Light Invocation*[26] which you might want to look up online on the Yasodhara Ashram website,[27] where you can also download an audio recording.

CHAPTER FIVE

Aparigraha

No longer attached
to people, things or outcomes.
Simple existence.

This chapter is centred round the concept of Aparigraha, which translates as non-grasping, non-possessiveness or non-attachment. It usually has a particular focus on material possessions, but it can also relate to people, situations and even the environment.

In this context, I relate it to compassionate presence, and the cultivation of a healthy non-attachment – of self or ego – to the outcomes of the work that you do with people living with cancer. It is so easy to get personally caught up in another's experience of suffering, and to hold oneself to some unrealistic or egoic expectation of *making things better.*

Let's be clear that *non-attachment* does not mean *detachment, disinterest or lack of concern.* Far from it; a healthy non-attachment is offered in the context of compassion and love. And so, the practices in this chapter offer a process and practice for the cultivation (Bhavana) of compassion, presence and loving kindness (Metta) for yourself and for the people you work with.

Cultivating compassion
What is compassion?

■ **QUESTION FOR REFLECTION**

Take some time to consider and maybe make notes on what you believe compassion to be, and also what compassion is not. You may wish to look up some definitions of compassion on the internet or in a dictionary, and then perhaps definitions of compassion from Buddhist and other religious perspectives.

Now, you might think it should come easily to work with people living with cancer from the heart of compassion, that it is the most obvious thing in the world that we would be compassionate towards someone who is suffering in body, mind or spirit. Perhaps so. But the idea of what it means to offer compassion requires a little more fleshing out. Sometimes, what we believe is compassion is actually coming from some other motivation such as sympathy, or the desire to rescue or help, or feeling somatic empathy (you feel their pain), or any other deeply rooted psychological reasons why we choose to do this work.

None of these things are wrong, but ultimately, without a healthy practice of compassionate presence, these motivations could easily lead to compassion fatigue and burnout. The section on the 'wounded healer' in Chapter Three offered some reflections for you to examine your own motivations behind your desire to help.

Compassion is an innate human experience, but it is also a practice, something that we can cultivate and develop. Compassion is not about feeling sorry for someone. In many ways that is easy to do. Compassion is about offering unconditional love and acceptance to the whole person, and feeling empathy with their suffering *without attachment*. Deeper than that, when we work from the heart of compassion, we aim to offer compassion to everyone, *starting with ourselves* and including those whose actions and behaviours we do not like. This is a tough call, but absolutely essential if we choose to follow the path of helping.

Metta (loving kindness)

There are exercises in the Buddhist tradition that allow us to focus on love and compassion in our meditation. The Loving Kindness meditation, or Metta Bhavana, begins the practices of the four Brahma-Viharas or 'sublime abodes'. These are:

- Metta Bhavana, the cultivation of loving kindness.

- Karuna Bhavana, the cultivation of compassion.

- Mudita Bhavana, the cultivation of sympathetic joy.

- Upekkha Bhavana, the cultivation of equanimity.

Metta is most often translated as 'loving kindness', but it can also be translated as friendliness, goodwill, benevolence, fellowship, amity and concord. Bhavana means to cultivate or establish. The Metta Bhavana allows the practitioner to begin to work with these practices in a gentle, but powerful, way. We only move on to the Karuna Bhavana, and then the subsequent practices, when Metta is deeply cultivated.

Metta usually involves the inward repetition of key phrases, but it can also be done by focusing on the feeling or awareness of loving kindness. In both, the idea is to begin by offering love to yourself, and then extending it outwards.

In the Metta Bhavana you practise offering loving kindness in this order, to:

1. Yourself.

2. Someone you care about.

3. Someone neutral, for example, an acquaintance of someone you know only in passing, someone you don't have any particular feelings about.

4. Someone with whom you have a difficult relationship.

5. Outwards from your immediate surroundings, gradually to encompass all sentient beings.

To practise Metta Bhavana: sit in your most comfortable seated pose for meditation. Make sure that your spine is long and your chest is open and that you can breathe easily. Take a few moments to focus on your breathing. Be aware of each breath as it arises, and allow other thoughts to drift in and out of your mind, coming back to your awareness of the breath any time your mind wanders.

1. Offering loving kindness to yourself: Bring your awareness to yourself in the spirit of loving kindness. Perhaps hold an image or an awareness of yourself in your heart space (Anahata). Offer yourself loving kindness. You can repeat inwardly these phrases:

   May I be happy.

   May I be safe.

   May I be healthy.

   May I be peaceful.

2. Offering loving kindness to someone you care about: May you be happy, etc.

3. Offering loving kindness to someone neutral.

4. Offering loving kindness to someone with whom you have a difficult relationship.

5. Offering loving kindness outwards to all sentient beings.

I always complete the cycle by coming back to offering loving kindness to myself. This is not the usual practice, but it feels appropriate to my practice.

There are many other wordings – short and long – that can be used to practice Metta Bhavana.

EXERCISE

You may wish to do some internet research on some alternative wordings for the Metta Bhavana.

Cultivating presence

As we explored in the section on the 'wounded healer' in Chapter Three, many people are drawn to working with people with cancer or other long-term conditions because of their desire to help or to 'give something back'. This is often the case when people have had a personal experience of a life-threatening diagnosis, or when they have lost someone close to them. This is a perfectly understandable desire, to offer something that can be of great help to others who need it. I spend a lot of time talking about this with my students, even before they are accepted on the Healing Space course. It is important that whoever chooses to do this work is ready to acknowledge the shadow side of rescuer and move into the role of offering their compassionate presence.

Yoga teachers are not there to fix people, but fixing is not always an easy thing to let go of. In my work as a mentor to new and student yoga teachers, I come across this a lot: the desire to make people better. And yet this desire comes from the need for us to feel better about someone else's pain or suffering, or to change something you have no control over. It is a difficult exercise, learning to bear witness without always feeling the need to offer solutions.

'Presence' is another word with diverse meanings. It has connotations of ego and charisma, but in this context, it means something quite different. Being present for someone is about being fully there and available to the presence of the other, however that manifests, even if it is in ways that you might ordinarily find uncomfortable. It may be difficult to witness someone else's distress without feeling that you need to do something to make it better for them. Working with compassion is one of the greatest features of this way of working. Whatever you offer, you can learn to work from the heart of compassion and not from your own desire to be free of distress. A witness to someone else's experience can never be sure that what they perceive in another is what they are actually experiencing. The only certainty is that it will change, because everything does.

This can be a difficult thing to unravel, and this is why I advocate a reflective practice in this work. Compassionate presence does not mean that you don't do anything to help. Yoga has the potential to be a deeply healing practice. In offering it in the full spirit of compassion, it can then become about bearing witness to the other person's experience as they are experiencing it, not how you might perceive or wish it to be.

So how do you offer your presence? At the heart of learning to be present, if indeed presence can be learned, is your own practice of yoga. Meditation offers the ability to be present, with awareness, to whatever is happening. It also develops the skill of being fully present to another. I always prepare myself in this way before I work with people. This is true in any context, whether it is a group class, a one-to-one yoga lesson or a therapeutic encounter. But it is particularly true in supporting those who are experiencing cancer or other life-threatening events.

Bearing witness

In her book *Being with Dying*[28] Joan Halifax includes a challenging, but wonderful, exercise in 'Bearing Witness', which I include in all my Yoga for Cancer training. I highly recommend reading the book and trying out the exercise for yourself.

Bearing witness is the practice of being present to someone else's experience in loving compassionate presence, without following the urge to fix, heal, control or change anything.

This does not mean that you detach or switch off from the suffering of another human being. Neither does it mean that you don't do anything. It means that you allow yourself to be fully and compassionately present to another's experience *as it is*, in a way that is validating to them, because there is no attempt in you to make it different in order to make it more comfortable for you to witness.

EXERCISE

The next time you have a conversation with a friend or a loved one who is going through some difficulty or who wants to let off some steam, I invite you to practise bearing witness to them in the spirit of your full presence. This means that you listen without interjecting, commenting or offering advice. Notice how it feels, for you and for them, to be able to be fully present – to really hear them – in this way.

Poetry

I love poetry and I use it a lot in my classes and one-to-one work. My belief is that poetry can help people connect to feelings and concepts in a way that simply talking cannot. The poet David Whyte speaks about poetry as saying the unsayable, in that it can speak of emotion in a way that isn't directly challenging or exposing, that crosses between the universal and the personal.

Poetry can also be a way of speaking about fear, pain or grief in a way that isn't simply about offering platitudes. There are many poets I call on, but among my favourites are John O'Donohue,[29] Mary Oliver[30] and David Whyte.[31]

EXERCISE

Start to gather your own collection of poetry, words, quotes and readings that you might use with your clients. I highly recommend the website, Poetry Chaikhana.[32]

CHAPTER SIX

Saucha

Practise clarity
in body, energy, mind.
Cultivate self-care.

In this chapter we explore the yogic view – from the perspectives of the Koshas, the Gunas and Ayurveda – of health and dis-ease. I chose to include them in the Saucha chapter, not because I had nowhere else to put them, but because Saucha – which translates as purity, cleanliness or clarity – relates very well to the yogic view of health being a mind/body/spirit affair. The focus is the *whole* person, rather than just their cancer.

I want to be explicit in my intention here, however, as especially the concept of purity – in any spiritual or physical tradition – can have extremely unhealthy, judgemental and triggering connotations. For that reason, I choose to use *clarity* as my primary translation of Saucha. Clarity is a spacious concept that invites curiosity, awareness and discernment. In this spirit, this chapter explores cancer from the traditional yoga perspectives, so that it might inform your process of creating and recommending appropriate practices for students that are embedded in yoga, as well as modern medical understandings.

The five Koshas

In yoga, the traditional view is that the soul (Atman) is covered in five (Pancha) layers or sheaths (Koshas). Yoga therapists view the manifestation and treatment of disease, including cancer, partly from the perspective of the Koshas, the belief being that when something is out of balance or there is a lack of integration in the Koshas, this creates imbalance in the system, thus causing dis-ease. Healing comes from reintegration, which results from the various practices of yoga.

The five (Pancha) Koshas are:

- Annamayakosha, the physical sheath.

- Pranamayakosha, the energy sheath.

- Manamayakosha, the mental or emotional sheath.

- Vijnanamayakosha, the wisdom sheath.

- Anandamayakosha, the bliss sheath.

Annamayakosha, the physical sheath
Anna = food; Maya = appearance.

Annamayakosha is the food sheath, our physical body, which is literally nourished by the food we eat. The physical body is the part of our experience to which we most relate, and it is generally the starting point of a yoga practice through Asana. For some practitioners, it might also include diet and fasting. All medicines prescribed in modern (Western) medicine tradition are said to act on this Kosha.

From the perspective of cancer treatment, the Annamayakosha may be affected in the following ways:

- Musculoskeletal system may be weakened due to treatment, protective posture and/or lack of activity.

- Immune system may be impaired due to treatment that results in the decrease of red and/or white blood cells.

- Respiratory system may be affected by the reduction in red blood cells, by tumours or by treatments.

- Nervous system effects may include exhaustion, confusion, forgetfulness, lability and insomnia.

- Endocrine system effects may include hormonal imbalances and menstrual disorders, including menopause induced by treatments.

- Digestive system effects may include nausea, vomiting, diarrhoea and decreased absorption of nutrients.

- Circulatory system: there may be a decrease in red and/or white blood cells, weakened blood vessels, anaemia.

- Reproductive system: there may be permanent or temporary infertility.

Pranamayakosha, the energy sheath

Prana = energy.

Pranamayakosha is the energy sheath, the sheath of Prana or life force. This is the energy that flows through and in everything.

In yoga we experience this vital energy most directly through the breath. Our practice of breath awareness and the breathing techniques of Pranayama tend to be the ways in which we engage with this vital flow of Prana.

The Nadis (energy channels) are thought to be located in the Pranamayakosha, as are the five organs of action (hands, feet, organ of speech, organs of evacuation and the organ of generation).

Effects of cancer treatment in the Pranamayakosha might include:

- Low energy level.

- Lack of breath awareness.

- Depression or anxiety.

- Separation at the level of the Chakras:

  - Muladhara: separation from the Earth, resulting in feelings of insecurity and not being grounded.

  - Swadisthana: separation from the senses and one's sexuality.

  - Manipura: separation from a sense of personal power.

- Anahata: separation from loving relationships.

- Vishuddha: separation from wisdom, inability to communicate clearly one's needs.

- Ajna: separation from one's spiritual nature.

Manamayakosha, the mental or emotional sheath
Manas = mind.

The Manamayakosha is the sheath of the mind and emotions and of the five senses. We tend to process our sensory experiences through the filter of the mind. This Kosha is also considered to govern the experiences of the Annamaya and Pranayama Koshas.

Effects of cancer treatment in the Manamayakosha include:

- Fear, particularly fear of death and fear for the wellbeing of children or dependants.

- Anger.

- Depression.

- Anxiety about the future.

- Despair and hopelessness.

- Shame about changes in appearance, e.g. hair loss.

- Loneliness.

- Guilt about distress of loved ones.

- Too much Rajas – 'doing too much'.

- Too much Tamas – inertia, not taking care of the self physically, emotionally, mentally or spiritually.

Vijnanamayakosha, the wisdom sheath
Vijnana = knowing.

Vijnanamayakosha is considered part of the subtle body and represents the higher mind, the faculty of wisdom, which lies underneath the processing, thinking, reactive mind. This is the level of our being that has the wisdom to guide us through life and lead us to higher and higher levels of truth and integration. It represents the reflective aspects of our consciousness, which allow us to experience a deeper insight into ourselves and the world around us. Meditation is considered to work at the level of the Vijnanamayakosha.

Effects of cancer treatment in the Vijnanamayakosha include asking questions such as 'Why did this happen to me?' and exploration of meaning in relation to the cancer diagnosis.

Anandamayakosha, the bliss sheath
Ananda = bliss.

Anandamayakosha refers not to a sense of transient happiness, but to the unbounded state of peace, joy and love that exists at the deepest level of our being. It is the layer closest to Atman, the self or soul at the deep heart of our being. Deep sleep or the state of awareness that we achieve in Yoga Nidra are considered to be the only ways to truly access the fullest expression of this sheath.

Effects of cancer treatment in the Anandamayakosha include an inability to be at peace with one's illness and the separation of not knowing the true essence of one's being.

QUESTION FOR REFLECTION
How does this model relate to modern scientific thinking about cancer?

The three Gunas
In the Samkhya school of thought, Prakriti (the material principle of nature) is considered to be made of three qualities, the three Gunas – Tamas, Rajas and Sattva – which exist in a state of equilibrium. Prakriti is said to become active, and creation takes place (evolution, the cycle of birth and death) when the Gunas lose their equilibrium. The Gunas, therefore, are both the cause of creation and the inherent qualities of all that is created. Everything is under the influence of these Gunas. And *we* are under the influence of these Gunas: our thoughts, actions, attitudes, motivations and influences.

Qualities of Tamas

- Darkness
- Inertia
- Inactivity
- Laziness
- Disgust
- Attachment
- Depression
- Helplessness
- Doubt
- Guilt
- Shame
- Boredom
- Addiction
- Hurt
- Sadness
- Apathy
- Confusion
- Grief
- Dependency
- Ignorance.

Qualities of Rajas

- Energy
- Action
- Change
- Movement
- Attraction
- Longing
- Attachment
- Anger
- Euphoria
- Anxiety
- Fear
- Irritation
- Worry
- Restlessness
- Stress
- Courage
- Rumination
- Determination
- Chaos.

Qualities of Sattva

- Harmony
- Balance
- Joy
- Intelligence
- Delight
- Happiness
- Peace
- Wellness
- Freedom
- Love
- Compassion
- Equanimity
- Empathy
- Friendliness
- Focus
- Self-control
- Satisfaction
- Trust
- Fulfilment
- Calmness
- Bliss
- Gratitude
- Fearlessness
- Selflessness.

Sattva is the state of balance and good health. According to Ayurveda and yoga, illness is caused by a disturbance in the Gunas – usually excessive Rajas or Tamas. In this school of thought, the development of cancer is thought to be related to an imbalance of or too much Tamas. The practices of yoga are supposed to cultivate the qualities of Sattva and counteract the imbalances of Rajas and Tamas that contribute to lack of wellbeing. This includes our diet. A yogic diet is a Sattvic diet.

QUESTIONS FOR REFLECTION

Looking at the various qualities of the three Gunas, how do the practices of yoga contribute to the cultivation of Sattva? How does this model relate to modern scientific thinking?

Ayurveda

We can also look at the development and treatment of cancer from the perspective of Ayurveda. Ayurveda is the ancient Indian practice of traditional medicine, which uses yoga as one of its healing disciplines.

Ayur = science/knowledge; Veda = Life.

The practice of Ayurveda is a rich and complex system and we can only briefly touch on it here. Whilst there is very little modern scientific evidence to support the efficacy of Ayurvedic medicines for the treatment of cancer, we do know that yoga – an aspect of Ayurveda – does have some efficacy as a complementary therapy, and thus Ayurveda provides a useful model for us to understand, if we are offering Yoga for Cancer. This brief discussion in no way qualifies you to treat anyone from an Ayurvedic perspective. For this, I recommend additional training or referral to an Ayurvedic practitioner. But it will help you to give yoga practices that will be of benefit.

We will look specifically at the three constitutional types or Doshas – Vata, Pitta and Kapha – and the five elements – Earth, Air, Fire, Water, Ether – and how Ayurveda views the manifestation of disease, especially cancer.

The three Doshas of Ayurveda

Each Dosha has its own qualities. One Ayurvedic perspective suggests that each person is considered to be naturally, and predominantly, one, or a combination of two, of these constitutions whilst another perspective suggests that in order for a person to be healthy, their Doshas should be perfectly balanced, the idea being that when a Dosha is out of balance, this is what manifests in dis-ease. Ayurveda is an holistic practice, and thus sees body, mind and spirit as one entity.

Vata – Air

The Vata qualities are movement, coolness and air. Vata is linked with the nervous system. Vata type people are 'airy', quick moving and often of slim build, with dry hair and skin. Vatas are quick thinking and imaginative. They have a tendency to chronic fatigue and burnout.

Pitta – Fire/Water

In contrast to Vata's dryness, Pitta is warm and moist. Pitta is linked to the metabolism. Pitta types are often hot and quick to becoming overheated. They are fiery, motivated and ambitious, but get easily frustrated.

Kapha – Earth/Water

Kapha energy is slow, steady, cool and heavy. Kapha is linked to the chest. Kapha people may have a tendency to hold onto extra weight. They have thick or curly hair and oily skin. They are slow moving, solid and dependable, and not very fond of change.

Ayurveda and tumours

From an Ayurveda perspective, tumours develop out of the relationship between Vata and Kapha. The erratic cell division we see in cancer is considered to be Vata, whilst the growth of these cells to form tumour sites is considered to be Kapha. The resulting cancer spread is an interplay of the two. A benign tumour is considered to be more Kapha. The inflammatory nature of some conditions also implicates Pitta. In yogic terms, we would consider this the Agni – the digestive fire – effectively turning on the body.

Gulma

Ayurveda refers to more than one type of condition – including cancerous tumours – as Gulma. Gulma usually refers to cancers that appear in the abdominal region, and is said to arise out of aggravated Vata. There are eight basic types of Gulma, relating to all three Doshas, their combinations and tridoshic types, and one relating to disorders of the Artava (diseases of the female organs). The word often refers simply to menstrual blood.

Symptoms of Vataja Gulma

- Tumours in the large intestine or pelvic region.

- Pain in the neck or head.

- Constipation.

- Dry skin.

- Dry mouth.

- Weight loss.

- Darkening or greying of the skin, nails, eyes, faeces.

- Cutting pain.

- Symptoms worse with empty stomach and at Vata times of day.

Symptoms of Pittaja Gulma

- Tumours in the small intestine or solar plexus.

- Hyperacidity and diarrhoea.

- Fever.

- Yellowing of the skin, nails, eyes and faeces.

- Burning pain – worse during the Pitta times of day and shortly after eating as food is digesting.

Symptoms of Kaphaja Gulma

- Tumours in the chest or stomach.

- Loss of appetite and nausea.

- Feeling cold.

- Whitening of skin, nails, eyes and urine.

- Tumour is slow growing, deep, hard, heavy and non-mobile.

- Little pain.

- Symptoms are worse during Kapha times and immediately after eating.

Symptoms of Raktaja Gulma (in women)
Raktaja is a tumour arising from the blood in the Artavavaha Srota and occurs only in women. Symptoms include:

- Ovarian cysts and uterine fibroids.

- Excessive menstrual bleeding.

- Anaemia.

- Fatigue.

- Abdominal swelling (before the days of scanning, it would have been difficult to tell sometimes if the woman was pregnant or not).

Dual Dosha and tridoshic Gulma combines the symptoms of the involved Dosha.

Practices for the Doshas
For Vata Dosha or a Vata imbalance, choose yoga practices that are:

- Calming

- Grounding

- Slow

- Warming
- Balancing
- Offer long relaxation.

For Pitta Dosha or Pitta imbalance, choose yoga practices that are:

- Calming
- Cool and cooling
- Balancing
- Breath-centred.

For Kapha Dosha or Kapha imbalance, choose practices that are:

- Stimulating
- Warming or heating
- Energizing
- Invigorating.

■ QUESTION FOR REFLECTION

Choose one (or all) of the Doshas, and based on these recommendations, think of practices (Asana, Pranayama, relaxation) that you might offer to someone who had a seeming imbalance of this Dosha.

For more in-depth information on Dosha-related practices I recommend Mukunda Stiles' book, *Ayurvedic Yoga Therapy*.[33]

CHAPTER SEVEN

Santosha

How to be happy:
When I practise contentment,
I become happy.

In this chapter, the container is Santosha, which translates as contentment, or the state of inner peace. And in this context it is considered a practice, that is, something that can be cultivated. So I have chosen to focus, in this chapter, on the various practices in yoga that are specific to cultivating a peaceful state of mind.

What we know without any doubt is that yoga is really good at helping people manage their stress. Indeed, when we are promoting the benefits of Yoga for Cancer, this is where there is the most scientific evidence. Even without the science, we know this just because we practise yoga and we know that it works!

So, we start the chapter with a look at cancer-related stress and a review of the stress response, the functions of the autonomic nervous system and evidence relating to the vagus nerve and vagal tone. Then we look in depth at the practices of meditation, relaxation and Yoga Nidra. Each of these sections contains specific practices that I have found particularly helpful in my work with people going through cancer treatment.

Yoga, cancer and stress

Stress is the body's natural response to pressure. And some stress is good. The body responds to stress through 'flight or fight', a physiological reaction that occurs when we perceive a threat. In the case of cancer, this threat is a life-threatening illness. It isn't a tiger at the mouth of the cave, but essentially the body perceives the threat of cancer in exactly the same way.

The fight or flight response might more accurately be described as the fight, flight, freeze or fold response (FFFF). The reactions that cause someone to collapse or become immobile in response to stress or trauma are just as likely as the impulses to fight or to run away. The archetypal 'bunny in the headlights' is a good example of the freeze response in a mammal that has swiftly and instinctively concluded it can neither fight the oncoming vehicle nor run fast enough to get away from it. Prey animals often display the 'fold' response when being outrun by predators. They collapse, as if dead, before they are actually caught. This has the benefit of making the animal appear dead and therefore less attractive to a predator that catches live prey, and also – because of the hormonal chemicals released – of making any subsequent attack less painful. As we are also mammals, we too have the capacity to respond to traumatic events – like a diagnosis of cancer – by freezing, or shutting down. When someone appears to have numbed out, or dissociated, this may be a natural protective, biological reaction to trauma.

What most mammals do, however, that we as humans appear to have lost the instinctive capacity for, is *shaking off* the trauma. You can observe this in your family dog. If the dog gets a fright, or even if you do something to annoy it, it will pause, then shake its body all the way from nose to tail. Hunted animals that manage to escape will display an extended period of trembling and shaking before returning to normal behaviour. This response is inbuilt. However, humans seem to have lost this innate capacity. Biologically, we are more likely to hang onto the effects of traumatic or stressful events in our bodies.

This FFFF response is a feature of the sympathetic nervous system (a branch of the autonomic nervous system) resulting in the release of the stress hormones adrenaline and noradrenaline. The release of these hormones is what stimulates the production of cortisol. Cortisol increases blood pressure and blood sugar, and suppresses the immune system. It also primes us to use available energy stores in the body, preparing the muscles to fight or to run away.

Symptoms of this release of hormones in the fight or flight response can include:

- Fast heartbeat.

- Quicker breathing.

- Going pale or becoming flushed.

- Sweating – especially the palms.

- Blood supply focused on the muscles and constricted elsewhere.

- Inhibited digestion.

- Dry mouth.

- Dilation of the pupils.

- Relaxation of the bladder.

- Restricted hearing.

- Tunnel vision (loss of peripheral vision).

- Shaking or tremor.

The parasympathetic nervous system, sometimes called the 'rest and digest' system, is the part of the autonomic nervous system that activates the return to normal after the fight or flight response. This system causes the release of the neurotransmitter acetylcholine.

The autonomic nervous system is always working; it isn't only active during fight or flight or rest and digest situations. Rather, the autonomic nervous system acts to maintain normal bodily function all the time.

We have already seen – in the section on the evidence-based science in Chapter Two – how yoga helps dampen the body's stress response by reducing levels of the hormone cortisol. Yoga also boosts levels of feel-good brain chemicals such as GABA, serotonin and dopamine. And as well as mediating the stress response, yoga also directly stimulates the parasympathetic nervous system. It lowers our heart rate and blood pressure, restores blood supply to the digestive organs, relaxes the muscles, and basically calms us down.

Vagal tone

Yoga also helps to regulate the nervous system by increasing what is called vagal tone, or the body's ability to respond successfully to stress. Vagal tone relates to the vagus nerve, our largest cranial nerve, which regulates breathing, heart rate and digestion, and directly influences activation of the sympathetic nervous system. People with healthy vagus nerve functioning are considered to have 'high vagal tone', meaning that their bodies and brains are more resilient under stress. People with low vagal tone, on the other hand, are more sensitive to stress and disease.

We know, through an increasing body of research, that the breathing techniques of Pranayama can significantly increase vagal tone. 'Resistance breathing', such as Ujjayi breathing, increases parasympathetic activity.[34]

■ QUESTION FOR REFLECTION

What yoga practices do you think are particularly useful for invoking the parasympathetic response?

Meditation

Meditation is a practice that is common to many mystical traditions. Nowadays, we most readily associate it with yogis and Buddhists, but pretty much every spiritual tradition has its own way of going inward, stilling the mind, and practising with attention or intention. Because it is associated with Eastern mysticism, some people feel that it must be inaccessible to them or that that it will involve chanting, or require them to sit crossed legged on the floor! I also think this is because there is some idea that it involves 'emptying' the mind. Any of us with a regular meditation practice know that this is simply not the case. The mind is never empty. But we can learn not to be too bothered by it.

Offering someone living with cancer some very simple meditation techniques can be incredibly helpful and empowering, because the basics are relatively easy to pick up and take away. And it requires nothing except a little space and time and something comfortable to sit on. There is no 'right' way to do meditation; there is only the way that works for the individual. Essentially at the heart of any meditation practice is the desire to come into stillness and awareness – stillness in the body, breath and mind, and awareness of *what is*. Some techniques are more intentional than attentional, and have a very particular focus such as contemplating a particular word or passage of scripture or practising Japa (repetition of a mantra) for a specific outcome. In this section, we look at a few techniques for accessing meditation.

Mindfulness

Much is spoken about mindfulness these days. It has become a very popular practice, which is now being integrated into mainstream psychology. This is largely due to the work of Jon Kabat-Zinn, who developed Mindfulness-Based Stress Reduction (MBSR). Because of his work, mindfulness practitioners are being trained to offer these techniques in a diverse range of settings. Mindfulness is a secular practice that draws its practical techniques from Buddhist Vipassana meditation and has a huge crossover with the practices of yoga. Indeed, another word for mindfulness might well be 'yoga'.

At the heart of the practice is the idea of being in full 'present moment' awareness. When we practise mindfulness, we are allowing ourselves to be with each moment as it arises. This can be in mindful awareness of our breathing, of our bodily sensations, of the input from our senses, of our thoughts as they come and go. And as we pay attention, we allow each awareness to pass through, without creating a narrative about it or making any judgement about it.

I have found the mindfulness practice of breath awareness to be one of the most valuable and powerful practices we can offer people living with cancer. Breath awareness is, of course, also a yogic practice. In yoga, we work with the body, breath, sensory withdrawal, one-pointed focus, attention and meditation, all of which are contained with the mindfulness practice.

Breath awareness

1. Sit in a comfortable position. Breathe gently through your nostrils and simply watch your breath for a while, without changing it in any way. You can focus on the sensation of your breath or on the sound it makes, or you can visualize the breath – whatever works for you. Through this, you may discover some aspect of your breath that creates a focus, or 'anchor' for you to come back to when your mind wanders.

2. After a while, you may begin to notice your breath naturally lengthening and deepening, but don't force this. Keep watching your breath. With ease. No judgement. Just noticing each breath as it arises. If your mind strays to other thoughts, gently guide it back to your anchor in the breath. Be gentle with yourself. You may feel frustrated when your mind wanders. This is part of the practice. Notice it. Let it go. Come back to your awareness of the breath.

Heart Chakra meditation

1. Start with breath awareness. Place the right palm in the centre of your chest (Anahata Chakra, the heart centre) and the left hand on top of the right. Close your eyes and feel the warmth and energy of your hands over your heart centre.

2. Now begin to visualize this energy as an emerald green light, radiating out from the centre of your heart into the rest of your body. Feel this energy flowing out into your arms and hands, and flowing back into the heart. Stay with this visualization for a few minutes.

3. When you feel full of beautiful heart Chakra energy, gently release the palms and turn them outwards with the elbows bent, shoulders relaxed and chest open. Feel or visualize the green light love energy flowing out of your palms and into the world. You can direct it towards specific loved ones in your life or to all sentient beings.

4. Finish by bringing your palms over the heart once more.

Body scan meditation

1. Allow your eyes to gently close or have a soft gaze. Feel the rising and falling of your belly with each inhalation and exhalation. Take a few moments to feel your body as a whole. Notice the points of contact between your body and the floor/bed/chair.

2. Now bring your awareness to the toes of your left foot. As you direct your attention to them, see if you can direct your breathing to them as well, so that it feels as if you are breathing into your toes and out from your toes. It may take a while for you to get the hang of this. And don't worry if you can't breathe into your toes; just allow your awareness to rest there. Allow yourself to feel any and all sensations in your toes. Try not to judge feelings as good, or bad, or to work out what it is you are feeling. Simply be aware. And don't worry if you don't feel anything – that's okay.

3. When you are ready to leave the toes and move on, take a deeper, more intentional breath in, all the way down to your toes and, on the out-breath, allow your toes to dissolve in your mind's eye. Stay with your breathing for a few breaths at least. Then move on in turn to the sole of your foot, your heel, the top of your foot and your ankle, continuing to breathe into and out from each region as you observe the sensations you are experiencing, and then letting go of that part of your body and moving on.

4. Continue to move slowly up your left leg and through the rest of your body. Stay with your focus on the breath and on the feeling of each body part as you come to it. Focus, breathe and then let go.

EXERCISE

Try other mindfulness practices.

Listen to the audio recordings of Mindfulness of Breathing and Mindfulness of Sound, which are among several excellent free downloads from Chris Germer.[35]

Also practise the Compassionate Body Scan Meditation from Dr Kristin Neff[36] at self-compassion.org, where there are also several excellent free downloads.

Relaxation

Relaxation is a powerful gift that yoga teachers can offer to people living with cancer. By learning to relax, the person experiences the feeling of allowing the tension in the body to dissolve, the mind to become less cluttered and the fear, pain or worry to subside, even if just for a short while.

For some people it will be the first time they have ever experienced relaxation. Some people will even say 'I can't relax' or 'I never relax'. I have rarely met anybody who genuinely *can't* relax if they are gently and sensitively guided through the process towards letting go. In my experience, it is often the people who have never experienced what relaxation feels like who respond most strongly to the practice. It can genuinely be a revelation.

Relaxation is taught in a wide range of contexts and involves a range of techniques, some of which have a crossover with yoga and some of which don't. At the heart of the practice of yoga is not relaxation as an end in itself, but rather the process of moving towards the state of awareness that *is* yoga – the awareness of our deepest self.

Technically, when we practise relaxation in yoga, we are not doing so through the use of external stimuli such as music or visualization of external images (places or situations external to our own inner experience), although these things can also be very helpful and are increasingly popular. Instead, the process is of moving through the layers of awareness. This can be seen almost as a process of unravelling or shedding.

The deepest way that we can practise this is through Yoga Nidra. Yoga Nidra is usually translated as 'yogic sleep', although it is actually a systematic process of achieving the brainwave state of deep sleep while still being consciously aware. (See the following section for a deeper exploration of Yoga Nidra.)

I have found it most useful to share other relaxation techniques: progressive muscle relaxation, spinal and body breathing techniques, a healing visualization technique called Body of Light, body scan meditation and Chakra meditations.

In yoga classes, relaxation techniques are typically done lying in *Savasana*. However, the most important thing about relaxing is that the person should be comfortable. They can lie in any position they want to, or sit. They should be encouraged to find the most comfortable position for them. You can help by making the surface that they are lying on as comfortable as possible, with pillows, blankets, cushions or any other supports that the person needs. Relaxation can be done lying or sitting in bed, or in a chair, depending on the person's individual needs. I often practise lying on my side because my back gets uncomfortable.

When using visualization techniques, consider the following:

- Not everyone is visual. Offer other sensory cues such as sensation or simply 'awareness of' so as not to exclude those who don't visualize easily.

- Exercise care around offering visualizations that involve specific locations or scenes, e.g. a beach or forest, unless you know that these places have relaxing connotations for your participants. A place, event or scene might just be a trigger for a traumatic memory. Stay neutral, or better, ask them what kinds of images, sounds or environments they find relaxing.

Progressive muscle relaxation

Progressive muscle relaxation (PMR) is the practice of systematically bringing attention to various parts of the body to consciously release tension, then noticing the feelings of softness and ease that arise. This can be a perfect experience for those who are habitually holding muscular tension that they may even be unaware of. In PMR we tense and contract the different parts of the body and then release, relax and let them go. Contractions are for about five seconds in the following order:

- Feet.

- Legs.

- Buttocks (clench).

- Abdomen and back (draw the lower back towards the floor).

- Shoulder blades (draw them together and lift the chest).

- Shoulders (hunch them up towards the ears).

- Arms (lift and tense).

- Hands and fingers (curl the fingers under tight, then spread them out wide).

- Face (squeeze the muscles of the face, then open the mouth and eyes wide and stick out the tongue).

Bear in mind that someone with a cancer diagnosis may find it uncomfortable, painful or even impossible to tense and release certain parts of their body in this technique, so be mindful of that when you are offering it.

Spinal breathing

This can actually be practised as quite an advanced Pranayama, but it can be simplified as a relaxation technique. The traditional practice involves breathing from the perineum to the third eye (point between the eyebrows), but I have modified the language to be less intimate. If the person is a more experienced practitioner, you can use the traditional language if you feel that is appropriate. It focuses the breath, allows the breath to become longer, and soothes and calms the nervous system.

1. Start with simple breath awareness.

2. Then begin to visualize, imagine or sense the breath moving

up and down the spine. As you inhale, feel the breath travel from the base of the spine to the crown of the head. As you exhale, feel the breath travel back down from the crown to the base of the spine.

3. Continue for a few minutes and then allow the breath to return to its natural rhythm, re-connecting with the sensations in the body and surroundings.

Body breathing

1. Start with simple breath awareness.

2. Then begin to visualize, imagine or sense the breath moving up and down the whole body. As you inhale, feel the breath travel from the soles of the feet all the way to the crown of the head. As you exhale, feel the breath travel back down from the crown to the soles of the feet.

3. Breathe like this for a few minutes, and then allow the breath to return to its natural rhythm, re-connecting with the sensations in the body and surroundings.

Body of Light

1. Start with simple breath awareness.

2. Begin to visualize/imagine that the breath is also energy and light. Imagine breathing this light into the heart centre.

3. Then begin to breathe the light out around the body. Imagine/visualize breathing in beautiful, radiant, healing light. Breathe it into your heart. And as you breathe out, breathe the light...

   a. Down into the legs and feet.

   b. Around the hips and pelvis.

   c. Abdomen and lower back.

   d. Chest, shoulders and upper back.

e. Arms, hands and fingers.

f. Neck and throat.

g. Face: mouth, tongue, jaw, eyes.

h. Forehead and scalp and inside of the head.

i. Around the whole body.

Option: visualize the light radiating outwards from the body like and aura.

4. Slowly come back into an awareness of breath, physical body and surroundings.

▨ QUESTION FOR REFLECTION

How do you think you might adapt these exercises for someone who was experiencing relaxation anxiety?

Yoga Nidra

There is probably no more powerful practice to offer a person living with cancer than Yoga Nidra. It is a deep and progressive way of relaxing the body and creating a very specific brainwave state. As mentioned in the last section, Yoga Nidra translates literally as 'yogic sleep', and indeed the practice takes you into a deep brainwave – theta or delta – state that is just like the state of deep rest or sleep, except than in Yoga Nidra, you remain awake.

There are four frequency ranges of waves that can be measured by an EEG (electroencephalogram):

- Beta waves: Show on an EEG when the person is awake, alert and actively processing information. They have a frequency range from 13–15 to 60 Hz. The range above 30–35 Hz is sometimes distinguished as gamma waves, which may be related to consciousness.

- Alpha waves: Usually found in people who are awake and alert but have their eyes closed and are relaxing or meditating. They have a frequency range from 8 to 12 Hz.

- Theta waves: Present during meditative, drowsy, hypnotic or sleeping states, but not during deep sleep. They have a frequency range from 3 to 8 Hz.

- Delta waves: Observed when individuals are in deep sleep or in a coma. Range from 0.5 to 3 or 4 Hz in frequency.

When there are no brain waves present, the EEG shows a flat-line trace, which is a clinical sign of brain death.

What is a Yoga Nidra practice?

There are a number of stages to the traditional Yoga Nidra practice, although these vary among different teachers. Indeed, many teachers of Yoga Nidra are taking the practice in wonderfully creative directions. What is typical about a Yoga Nidra practice, though, is that it is a systematic way of taking the body and mind into a deeper level of consciousness or awareness. These are the steps that I often follow when leading Yoga Nidra (although I also often talk through a shortened version).

1. Preparation

The first stage is setting up the space, the body and everything required to be comfortable and relaxed. Invite the student/client to practise Yoga Nidra, explain what it is and how it works and what is going to happen.

2. Relaxing the body

Introduce a short, led relaxation exercise to bring the body and mind into preparation for Yoga Nidra. Or (for more experienced practitioners) simply invite the student/client to relax.

3. Sankalpa (personal resolve)

Sankalpa is a much misunderstood concept. In the practice of yoga it translates as a vow, resolve or declaration of intention or purpose. I have observed it being confused with 'affirmation' and it isn't quite the same thing. I put it most simply, at the beginning of my yoga classes, by asking the students/clients to acknowledge what brought them to the mat that day. Essentially, 'Why are you here?'

In the context of yoga for people living with cancer, a useful and empowering guide to generating a Sankalpa can be found by inviting the person to acknowledge their body's (or heart's) deepest desire for healing or wholeness. It doesn't need to arrive in their awareness in words, or anything concrete. Simply the acknowledgement that the body has wisdom is enough. It has been the practice in certain schools of Yoga Nidra to be quite prescriptive about way a Sankalpa is and how it should be used. This creates stress, which is the opposite of Yoga Nidra. Nidra is a powerful, and radical, invitation to rest. The Sankalpa is merely an invitation to create intention.

4. Rotation of consciousness

Rotation of consciousness is a conscious mapping of the body, through a relatively swift, guided awareness of the physical body, taking awareness systematically to each different body part. In doing so we simultaneously 'map' the corresponding regions of the brain. In yogic terms, it contributes to the practice of Pratyahara, or withdrawal of the senses, and promotes a deep and relatively quick state of relaxation in the body and brain.

There are different ways to start and end the rotation of consciousness and different traditions offer different patterns and methodologies. There are many scripts online for you to explore, and I encourage you to experience as much Yoga Nidra as possible.

One of the techniques I like to use is a rotation similar to the '61 points' method, which is also known as Shavayatra.

The 61 points

1. Point between the eyebrows.

2. Centre of the throat.

3. Right shoulder.

4. Right elbow.

5. Right wrist.

6. Right thumb.

7. Index finger.

8. Middle finger.

9. Ring finger.

10. Little finger.

11. Wrist.

12. Elbow.

13. Shoulder.

14. Centre of the throat.

15. Heart centre.

16–27. Repeat steps 3–14 on the left.

28. Right side of the chest.

29. Heart centre.

30. Left side of the chest.

31. Heart centre.

32. Solar plexus.

33. Navel centre.

34. Right hip.

35. Right knee.

36. Right ankle.

37. Right big toe.

38. Second toe.

39. Third toe.

40. Fourth toe.

41. Fifth toe.

42. Right ankle.

43. Right knee.

44. Right hip.

45. Navel centre.

46–57. Repeat points 34–45 on the left side.

58. Solar plexus.

59. Heart centre.

60. Centre of the throat.

61. Point between the eyebrows.

5. Conscious breathing
Following the rotation of consciousness is an invitation to come back to the conscious awareness of the flow of the breath and an awareness of the body doing the breathing, or indeed, the breath breathing the body. It is at this point that you may notice some people appear to be asleep. This is okay. Trust that sleep is what is required, and that the Nidra will reach their awareness even so.

6. Exploring opposites
A very simple practice might involve moving between feelings of lightness and heaviness, heat and cold, or between the left and right sides of the body. It allows the mind to accept the possibilities of state change/altered state that allow for deeper receptivity to the practice. In some forms of Yoga Nidra, this might include an exploration of opposing emotional states. My feeling is that unless you have received deeper training in Yoga Nidra, then keep it to a simple exploration of sensation.

7. Visualization
In the more traditional styles of Yoga Nidra this would be a focus on the Chakras, for example the third eye, throat and heart. Modern versions of Yoga Nidra include more creative forms of guided imagery. I often use the 'Body of Light' visualization, or an adapted

version of it, in Yoga Nidra for people living with cancer, as it is powerful healing visualization that most people seem to respond to positively.

The techniques of visualization take the student into a place of creativity and receptivity. Visualizations can be spaces of healing, learning, journeying or receiving inner guidance. In all cases, it is important to be aware that in the practice of Yoga Nidra, the student is extremely vulnerable and open to suggestion, so what you suggest, as the teacher, can be powerful. The invitation is to enter into this role with great humility, and with the utmost ethical intention. As with all of the practices that you offer, gaining informed consent is important. It is always worth checking in with your student(s) about any proposed visualization technique, to make sure that it is going to land well, and that nobody is going to be triggered by it.

8. Repeat Sankalpa

As you begin to bring the students/clients out of the Yoga Nidra, and at this point of deepest receptivity, there is an invitation to repeat the Sankalpa, in words, or in intention.

9. Coming back to external awareness

At the end of the yoga practice, the student/client is guided out of the state of Yoga Nidra, gently and gradually to allow them to come back into full present moment awareness without feeling disoriented. Taking time with this part of the practice is important, as some people take longer to extricate themselves from Nidra than others (and I am one of them). It is also important that if you do a Yoga Nidra at the end of a session that there is enough time afterwards for people to ground themselves, and to feel safe enough to leave.

The best way to familiarize yourself with the practice is to do it as much as possible. For this I recommend the free recordings at the Yoga Nidra Network.[37] I also highly recommend the courses – including an introductory immersion course – offered by Uma Dinsmore Tuli and Nirlipta Tuli, of Total Yoga Nidra.[38]

CHAPTER EIGHT

Tapas

I become strong when
I commit to my practice.
Body, mind, senses.

At last, we come to the chapter that deals with the postures and breathing! If you've read this far, you'll know why I put it here, and not at the beginning. It is safe to say that in most yoga classes in the West, yoga has become synonymous with Asana, which is really only one aspect of the practice of Hatha Yoga, and a tiny aspect of all the other practices that can be described as yoga. Modern postural yoga – as it has become known – in many settings, really just looks like a sort of exercise class, maybe with a little breathing and meditation thrown in (although not always!).

If I ask non-yoga people what they think about yoga, they usually have an idea of someone doing some sort of posture or pose. And usually an improbable one, like putting your leg behind your head, or a handstand, or the splits. I really do wish I had a pound for the number of times I have been asked if I can do those things. I can't, I don't want to, and it doesn't make me less of a yogi or a yoga teacher because I can't.

As we know, Hatha Yoga is more than Asana. Hatha Yoga is a discipline of several practices that include Asana, Pranayama, Mudra, Mantra, Bandha and Kriya. In this chapter we focus specifically on the first four, which are included in this chapter about Tapas, meaning discipline, austerity or commitment. The practices of Hatha Yoga were always intended as a discipline, that is, something that the student is required to practise regularly to get any benefit. If the word 'discipline' makes you feel uncomfortable – and I can imagine why it might – it is likely that the word 'austerity' doesn't land any more comfortably. For this reason, I choose to define Tapas as 'commitment'.

Committing to the practices of Hatha Yoga does not mean that you need to commit yourself to a rigorous, unbending and uncomfortable discipline. In this context – of working with people living with cancer – I offer commitment as a way to engage with using the practices regularly and in a structured way to realize their benefits.

Essentially, it doesn't work if you don't do it!

Asana (posture)

Patañjali was most likely referring to the seated posture when he said that it should be both steady and comfortable. But the term Asana, certainly in modern postural yoga, has come to describe the range of postures that we employ in the practice of Hatha Yoga. This section deals with how we approach adapting the postural practices of Hatha Yoga for the physical needs and limitations of our students who are living with cancer. And in the process, potentially changing how we teach ALL of our students.

The Asana practice is where you may need to make the greatest modifications to the yoga practice for people living with cancer. You will be able to offer different things depending on how you are working with the person: in a general mixed class, in a one-to-one private session, or in a class specifically adapted for people with cancer. A major consideration is the person's general physical condition. This will determine where you start: whether the person is able to sit on the floor or whether you will need to adapt the practice to a chair.

In this section I offer four sample practices:

- A chair yoga class that can be offered to a mixed group of people living with cancer.

- A one-to-one practice designed around the needs of an individual.

- A restorative class specifically for a group of people living with cancer.

- Guidance on how to integrate people living with cancer into your general yoga classes.

These are provided, not as off-the-shelf trademarked sequences, but as a structure around which to reflect on how you might adapt to the case studies given, and to inform your own experimentation in your practice.

Why I don't offer any standard sequences

It would be the easiest thing in the world to give you a few sequences, and then say, off you go – teach this! But for several reasons, that is not what I am about. First, you already have your own teaching practice, style and way of teaching. You know how to teach, and I would love for you to keep teaching it with the new knowledge and skills that you learn in this book. This is how you learn to make the practice your own.

Second, there isn't a standard practice that I can give you for this work. Other books and courses may try, but the reality is, there will always be someone for whom that practice won't be suitable. Everyone is different, and every person with cancer is different. So the best thing that you can learn to do is adapt your practice to the needs of whoever shows up.

Finally, learning to do this work takes time and confidence. If I gave you a few scripts of classes to teach, this would not give you confidence, or indeed me confidence that you were happy to adapt to the person or the circumstances. The quality of my training is very important to me. This is literally my life's work. If I could download it to you Matrix-style, I would, but time is what it takes! I hope this, at the very least, gives you confidence in me as your teacher.

Conversation with gravity

In my experience, this feeling of connection to the Earth is fundamental to my embodied wellbeing. It is also my experience, through long years of teaching embodiment practices, especially to those who are unwell – in body, mind or spirit – that getting down on the floor or ground (or getting the feet onto the floor) and feeling into bodily connection to the Earth is a fundamental part of the practice of embodied wellbeing. It begins and finishes every one of my classes. So if I were to prescribe any aspect of a practice in Healing Space, it would be this.

Before I go any further, this is not about the concept of 'Earthing' or 'Grounding' – an idea about the transfer of electrons that some people think is pseudo-science (my jury is out). My take on this is about the *awareness* of connection. Walking barefoot, for example, increases our embodied awareness of being connected and it also enhances proprioception, which is considered to be our sixth sense, the ability to sense stimuli arising within the body regarding position, motion and equilibrium. This is why practising yoga barefoot – if it is physically safe and accessible – is a really good idea.

Whatever is going on physiologically, psychologically or energetically, being and feeling connected to the Earth has an immediately beneficial effect when someone is feeling scattered, stressed, disconnected, panicky or overwhelmed. I am my own guinea pig in this respect.

Opening sequence

This opening sequence begins all of the sample practices offered in this section.

1. Lie down comfortably. Perhaps bend your knees or place a bolster, pillow or rolled-up blanket under your knees. Or you might sit on a chair with your feet flat on the floor, or you may even be standing.

2. Sense that through the structure and foundation of the building, you are also connected to the Earth beneath.

3. Notice all the points of contact between you and the Earth: the feet/heels; backs of the legs; back; shoulder blades; arms; hands; back of the head. All settling more deeply into that connection. Setting up a conversation with gravity.

4. Take a deep breath in, and then sigh the breath out. Perhaps with sound. Do this three or four times.

5. Breathe naturally and let your awareness come to the natural flow, rhythm or sensation of your breath and the movement of your body as you breathe.

6. Come back into awareness of your body and its connection with the Earth. Be aware of your body, your breath and the sense of your body breathing.

7. When you are ready, and feeling grounded, bring your awareness back into the space around you.

Practising in a chair

If someone can get down on the floor (and back up again), consider inviting them to do that. The range of exercises, and the feeling of empowerment, can be greater. However, if someone is really un-well, or their mobility is particularly restricted, or they are extremely fatigued, or they just don't want to get down on to the floor, then practising in a chair might be just the right thing to do. It may be that you don't do the whole session in a chair, but you have it there just in case it is needed. It can be used to sit down on, or for support in standing postures.

The basic chair sequence offered here is based on Pawanmuk-tasana (the Joint Freeing Series), but it is possible to adapt any Asana to a chair if you are imaginative and willing to experiment in your own practice. I encourage you to do so.

The best type of chair for seated yoga is an upright dining or office-style chair with a back and no arm rests, and no wheels. The back rest allows you to place pillows or cushions behind the person's back, and the upright position means that nobody ends up slumping. However, you may have to adapt to whatever type of chair is available in the venue that you are in. It may be that the person is in a wheelchair, or requires a chair with arms for support.

Pawan means wind; Mukta means release; Asana, of course, re-lates to pose or posture. Thus, the Pawanmuktasana sequences are considered to release the flow of energy, removing any blockages that prevent its free flow in the body or mind. Generally, there are six repetitions of each exercise, but you may need to review this, depending on the energy levels of the participants. Although the exercises may seem – at first glance – quite easy, they can be taxing for some people who are unwell or fatigued. These exercises are easily adapted to people in wheelchairs or even lying in bed. And because they can give a feeling of working quite hard, they are useful for those who are frustrated that they cannot do their normal range of physical activity.

The following sequence is an adapted version of Pawanmuktasana, divided into three sections. Make sure to build in plenty of pauses for rest and to come back to the breath.

Start with the opening sequence outlined in 'Conversation with gravity' adapted to a chair.

1. Toe curls: Inhale, spread the toes out; exhale curl the toes under (x 6 on each side). Adapt in a chair by doing one leg at a time, right, then left.

2. Ankle flexion and extension: Inhale and point the toes; exhale and push the toes away (x 6 on each side).

3. Ankle rotation: Rotate the right ankle clockwise and then anti-clockwise (x 6 on each side).

4. Hip flexion/extension: Hold the right leg under the thigh and draw the knee gently up towards the chest (as far as is comfortable). Then, as you inhale, extend the leg away from you. Exhale and draw the knee towards the chest (x 6 on each side).

5. Cat/Cow: Sit with hands on your thighs. Exhale, tilt your pelvis gently backwards around the spine and let your hands slide forwards. Inhale, tilt the pelvis forwards, lift and open your chest, let the hands slide back and gently look up (x 6).

6. Wrist flexion/extension: Extend your arms with the hands palms down. As you inhale, raise your hands so that the fingers point upwards. As you exhale, point the fingers downwards (x 6).

7. Wrist rotations: Make soft fists and extend your arms.

Rotate your wrists three times in one direction and three times in the opposite direction (x 6).

8. Elbow flexion/extension: Extend your arms with the palms facing up. As you exhale, draw your fingertips towards your shoulders, bending at the elbow only. As you inhale, extend your arm outwards again (x 6).

9. Opening the chest and shoulders: Bring your fingertips to your shoulders and your elbows up to about mid chest height. As you exhale, draw your elbows towards each other. As you inhale, open them out wide, like wings (x 6).

10. Raised arms: As you inhale, reach your arms up. Lengthen from the sides of your waist into your fingertips and try to keep your shoulders from hunching up around your ears. Hold for three, four or five breaths.

11. Chest opener/shoulder stretch: Interlock your fingers and take your hands behind your back. Feel the shoulder blades squeeze towards each other. Your hands may lift away from your back, but don't let this curl your body forwards. Hold for three, four or five breaths.

12. Side stretch: Sit with your spine long and your right hand on the chair beside you. Inhale, and as you exhale gently bend to the right. Hold for three, four or five breaths. Repeat on the left.

13. Rotation of the spine: Sit with your spine long and your right hand on the chair beside or (if there is space) behind you. Inhale, and as you exhale gently twist around to the right. Hold for three, four or five breaths. Repeat on the left.

14. Neck flexion and extension: As you inhale, raise your chin and look up. As you exhale, draw your chin down towards the notch at the top of your chest (x 6).

15. Neck stretch: Sit erect. Inhale, then exhale and let your right ear come down towards your right shoulder. Hold for three,

four or five breaths. Inhale as you bring your head back to centre. Repeat on the left.

16. Head turns: Sit erect. Inhale, and then as you exhale, turn your head to the right. Inhale back to centre. Exhale and turn your head to the left (x 3 on each side).

EXERCISE

For the next few days, take your own Asana practice into a chair. See how you can adapt what you would normally do into a chair. Try different sorts of chairs to practise how you would adapt to being in a teaching environment where the 'right' sort of chair wasn't available. Experiment with using props – cushions, pillows, blocks under the feet, etc. Be imaginative and experimental. Have fun!

Working one to one

Ideally, all yoga classes would be one to one, as this is the best way to adapt a yoga practice to the specific needs and abilities of the individual. The sequence below is based on a 'standard' floor-based practice that I might try out with someone living with cancer, adapting as I go to their specific needs, offering modifications, props – blankets, cushions, pillows, bolsters, blocks, straps, etc. – as required.

In reality, there is no off-the-shelf yoga practice that I can offer you, because there is no off-the-shelf person! This practice is given as an example, based on a practice that I offered one of my real clients. It serves to give you some suggestions as to the kinds of things that might help you to explore gentle spinal movements, starting slowly and with awareness, to build up a sensitive picture of what might be available to the person. I pretty much start every class and one-to-one session I offer like this, on the floor. It helps to bring groundedness and awareness.

As with all physical practices, there are caveats based on injury, illness, side effects of treatment, etc. that will determine what practices you may and may not offer. But more often than not, if you go *slowly, gently and with awareness*, you can gently try things out, and then change them if they don't work. This is not to say that people going through cancer treatment can't do more challenging practices, because sometimes they can, and it might be what they want and need, but you need to know your client, and really feel into their needs and abilities – which may change every time you see them.

1. Start with the opening sequence outlined in 'Conversation with gravity'.

2. Bring both knees up towards your chest. Hold your shins, knees or thighs, and slowly and gently rock from side to side.

3. Bring your feet to the floor. Rock your knees from side to side, massaging over the hips, sacrum, lower back and sides of the buttocks.

4. Bring your right knee in. Draw it towards your chest as you exhale, and gently move it away from you as you inhale. Repeat this movement for a few breaths. Repeat on the left side.

5. Come up to sitting.

6. Shoulder stretches:

    a. Inhale and circle your arms above your head, exhale and lower them back down to your sides. Repeat a number of times, really connecting to the flow of your breath.

    b. Circle your arms above your head. Interlock your fingers, rotate your palms up and push the palms up towards the ceiling. Lengthen the back of your neck and lengthen up from the sides of your waist. Breathe deeply as you hold the stretch.

7. Side stretches: Take your right hand out to the side, palm flat on the floor, elbow a little bent. Raise your left arm as you inhale, and as you exhale, stretch it over your ear for a side stretch. Hold for a few breaths. Come up on an inhale. Repeat on the left.

    a. Take this side stretch into a flowing movement.

b. Inhale and raise the arm; exhale and stretch over to the side. Inhale and raise the arm back up; exhale and release. Then do the same on the other side.

8. Circle your shoulders: Move them up and back and down, inhaling as they come up, exhaling as they come down. Repeat a few times.

9. Come on to all fours: Bring your knees hip-width apart and under your hips, and your hands shoulder-width apart and under your shoulders, fingers spread. You may wish to place a folded blanket under your knees for support.

10. Cat/Cow: Exhale and draw your spine towards the ceiling, tail down and head down (looking back towards your thighs). Inhale and lift your tail, drop your belly, lift your chest and look forwards. Repeat to flow in time with your breath about six times.

11. Extended Child's Pose: Sit back towards your heels and stretch your arms forward. Breathe here for a while, feeling the expansion of the back of your ribs as you breathe and your spine lengthening out. Allow your shoulder blades to fall open. Stay in this pose for as long as you are comfortable. You may wish to take some deep breaths and sigh the breath out, finding release with each exhalation.

12. Modified Camel Pose: Come on to your knees, with your knees under your hips. Take a folded blanket under your knees for support. Place your hands on your lower back with the thumbs to the outside and the fingertips pushing down into the tops of your buttocks. Push forward into your hips/ thighs and lift/open your chest towards the ceiling. Keep your shoulders easy and relaxed. Open your heart/chest area. Breathe and feel the expansion in your side ribs.

13. Repeat extended Child's Pose.

14. Neck stretches – flexion/extension: Inhale and take your chin upwards. Exhale and bring your chin towards the notch at

the top of your chest. Feel the gentle muscle activation at the sides of your neck. Repeat three times, pausing on the third.

15. Neck stretches – rotation: Exhale to turn your head to look over your right shoulder. Inhale back to centre. Exhale to the left. Inhale back to centre. Repeat three times both sides.

16. Neck stretches – lateral flexion: Exhale and take your right ear towards your right shoulder. Keep your shoulders level and let gravity take over. Hold for a few gentle breaths. Repeat on the left.

17. Circle your shoulders again.

18. Come back into Savasana (a relaxation pose) for a relaxation.

EXERCISE

With the help of your research from organizations like Prostate Cancer UK,[39] make notes against each section about how you might need to modify or adapt a practice for someone with prostate cancer who has received a radical (retropubic) prostatectomy.

Radical retropubic prostatectomy is a surgical procedure in which the prostate gland is removed through an incision in the abdomen. It is most often used to treat individuals who have early prostate cancer. It can be associated with complications such as urinary incontinence and erectile dysfunction.

Restorative practice

I once read something that said restorative yoga is like nap time for grown-ups. It is a little like that, I suppose, but the intention is not just to rest, but to actively engage in practices that focus on restoring energy to the body, calming the nervous system, and either passively stretching or completely relaxing the muscles. A restorative Asana practice is about finding ways to be in poses, whilst eliminating, or at the very least, minimizing, effort. Often this requires the liberal use of props to support, elevate, soften, cushion, etc. We all know that the ubiquitous restorative yoga prop is the bolster!

Other props you might find useful:

- Block(s).

- Cushion(s).

- Bolster or pillows.

- Blankets – two or three are useful.

1. Start with the opening sequence outlined in 'Conversation with gravity'.

2. Bring both knees up towards your chest. Hold your shins, knees or thighs and slowly and gently rock from side to side. Bring your feet to the floor and rock your knees from side to side, massaging over the hips, sacrum, lower back and sides of the buttocks.

3. Bring your right knee in. Draw it towards your chest as you exhale, and gently move it away from you as you inhale. Repeat this movement for a few breaths. Repeat on the left side.

4. Roll over and gently push up to sitting.

5. Supported forward bend: You might want a folded blanket or cushion underneath your hips to gently tilt the pelvis. Place a rolled-up blanket under the knees so the knees can stay soft. Place a bolster on top of the thighs. Place a block on top of your bolster – either at the second or lowest height. Let the legs relax and rest the forehead on the block. Soften and release with each breath. Remain for up to five minutes, or as long as is comfortable and restful.

6. Legs up the wall: Place a bolster or two thickly folded blankets lengthwise along a wall, about 3 inches away from the wall. This creates a little lift in the pelvis and a soft support for the hips. Sit on the bolster or blanket sideways onto the wall. Swivel round and let the legs come up the wall and lie back. You might want to have something soft

under your head. Make any adjustments you need for it to be super comfy! Then, let the arms open, palms facing up toward the ceiling, in whatever position allows them to completely soften to the floor. You can remain in the pose for as long as it feels good! To come out of the pose, gently bend the knees and press the feet into the wall, lift your hips off the bolster and roll over on to one side.

7. Supported Child's Pose: Sit on your heels with a bolster (pillow, cushion or rolled-up blanket) lengthwise between the thighs. Fold forward on to a bolster (or two) with the head resting to one side. The arms can hug the bolster. A cushion or rolled-up blanket can also be placed under the buttocks (between the buttocks and the heels) and under the feet if required.

8. Supported Savasana (a relaxation pose): Lie down with your head supported and a pillow, bolster or rolled-up blanket under your knees. You can pad yourself out with cushions under your arms. Make it SUPER COMFY! You do not need to lie in the classic Savasana position – for example, you might lie on your side supported by a bolster or with a pillow between the knees.

9. Follow with a relaxation sequence.

EXERCISE

Have a look at the information on living with a colostomy from Colostomy UK[40] and from Macmillan.[41] Then reflect on how you might help to adapt this restorative practice for someone with a colostomy.

Integrating into a general yoga class
You may be reading this book because you already have a student in your class who has received a cancer diagnosis. It may be a long-term student who keeps coming to your class following their diagnosis, or someone new who has chosen to start a yoga practice because they have heard that yoga might help them. For all sorts of reasons,

not everyone wants to go to a special 'Yoga for Cancer' class, and there might not even be one available locally. Whatever the reasons, I encourage you not to turn this person away because you don't feel 'qualified'. I have heard this tale all too often. Hopefully, having got to this point in the book, you are beginning to feel a bit more confident that you can help to adapt a practice for almost anyone who comes through your door.

As with all of our practices, you will need to be prepared to make changes to your lesson plans for their specific needs, offering modifications, changes to the practice, props –blankets, cushions, pillows, bolsters, blocks, etc. – as required.

There are two main methods that I use to teach integrated classes that have become a standard part of my teaching practice for everyone. Both are based on the principle of choice.

'Tiering'

This means that for each practice that I offer, I start with the most accessible version of it that everyone can do, and then give two, three or four further options of increasing the challenge for those who can do those bits. In this way, you do not have to think of a special thing for the one person in the class who can't do what you had planned, as that leads to singling someone out, and they might feel embarrassed or vulnerable. For example, if I am teaching Tree Pose, I might offer the practice in this order:

1. (Everyone) Perhaps you want to try standing with the weight on your left foot and the toes of the foot on the floor. If you feel you need some help with balance today, then you might want to hold on to a chair or take support from the wall. (Notice that I give the invitation to everyone.)

2. You might want to see how it feels to take the foot with the toes on the floor to the inside of (a) the ankle or (b) the lower leg or (c) the inner thigh or (d) maybe you would prefer to keep the foot on the floor, or try it and bring the foot back to the floor when you need to.

3. How would it feel to try bringing the palms together in front of the chest? Remember – you can come back to the support of the chair or the wall at any time.

4. If you feel stable here, perhaps you might want to try raising the arms up towards the sky.

Invitational language

Invitational language gives people the option to try something, rather than giving an out and out instruction. Making a practice invitational and optional lets people know that everything you offer is a choice. This is at the heart of an accessible, integrated and trauma-aware practice.

Examples of invitational language:

- When you are ready...

- You might want to try...

- Perhaps you...

- Maybe you...

- How would it feel to...

- In your own time...

- Feel free to...

- You are welcome to experiment with...

EXERCISE

Look at information on lymphoedema following surgery for breast cancer. You can find this on the Breast Cancer Now website.[42] Now, take a lesson plan for a class you might normally teach. How would you adapt the exercises in this general yoga class for someone who has had breast surgery with lymph nodes removed from under the arm, and who is at risk of developing lymphoedema? What examples of invitational language might you use?

The breath
Cultivating a breathing practice
Take a deep breath!

Age old advice for someone who is feeling panicky. But yogis know, and science now agrees, that the wisdom is sound. Slow, deep breathing has a range of effects that help us to become calmer.

Working with the breath is one of the most direct, accessible and effective practices that we can use with people living with cancer. And it is always the starting point of any practice that I offer. In fact, it could be that this is the only thing you do with someone in a practice. Some practices will be more accessible than others, depending on how the person is, physically and emotionally. Before we begin looking at specific practices, let's examine briefly the anatomy and physiology of breathing. The organs of respiration are highlighted in bold.

The process of breathing (respiration) consists of the phases of inspiration (inhalation) and expiration (exhalation). When we inhale, the **diaphragm** contracts and pulls downward while the muscles between the ribs contract and pull upward. The size of the thoracic cavity increases and the pressure inside decreases. This causes the air to rush in and fill the **lungs**.

The air enters the body through the **nose or mouth**, travels down the throat through the **larynx** (voice box) and into the **trachea** (windpipe) before entering the lungs. The air is moistened and warmed before it reaches the lungs. When we exhale, the diaphragm relaxes, the volume of the thoracic cavity decreases, and the internal pressure increases. This causes the lungs to contract and the air to be forced out.

▦ QUESTIONS FOR REFLECTION

Think back to the section on the sympathetic and parasympathetic nervous systems (Chapter Seven). Why does slow, deep breathing have a calming effect?

As well as the obvious physiological effects, why else do you think yoga breathing techniques might help to calm the body and mind?

How to breathe
Simple breath awareness

Imagine working with someone who has never practised yoga before. And nobody has ever talked to them about breathing, or that there is maybe a healthy way to breathe. It is just something they take for granted. They breathe in, and they breathe out. Simple. This is the most likely scenario when you work with someone experiencing cancer. And so, you might have to – as the song goes – start from the very beginning. You might not want to start with a breathing 'technique' as such, but with an exercise that simply brings them into awareness of their breathing. In fact, this is the way I start all of my yoga classes, whether the students are experienced or not.

1. Sit comfortably in a chair, or lie down.

2. Let your eyes close, or a soft downward gaze, and feel the connection between your body and the chair and your feet on the floor.

3. Bring your awareness to your breathing. The naturally arising movement, sensation or rhythm of the breath as it enters and leaves the body.

4. Focus on whatever aspect of the breath you are most drawn to: it might be the movement of the belly or chest, or the sensation of the breath in the nostrils, or the sound. Simply notice the breath coming in and out of your body. And follow the breath.

5. Breathing in. Breathing out.

6. Following each breath as it arises.

7. When the mind wanders, gently guide yourself back to your awareness of the breath.

8. Continue for a while until you begin to feel more settled, then open your eyes or lift your gaze.

Note: This exercise does not instruct the person to breathe in any particular way. It is simply about connecting with the breath. What

I find is that just being aware of the breath makes it deeper and more regular, but this is not our goal here. We don't want to make people feel wrong; we just want to help them find their breath and to focus the mind.

Abdominal (belly) breathing

Abdominal breathing is about freeing up the belly to begin to access the full capacity of the breath. For some people who have not practised any form of breathing technique before, this might be where you need to start. It is from learning this practice that we can move on to the other breathing exercises. This way of breathing also makes meditation much more accessible, as it teaches a deeper, longer and less stressful way of breathing.

The diaphragm is a large, dome-shaped muscle located at the base of the lungs. The abdominal muscles help move the diaphragm. And learning how to free up the belly can help people learn how to free up the diaphragm, which ultimately makes it easier to breathe, especially if someone has breathing difficulties relating to lung disease or their treatment.

Abdominal breathing is most easily done lying down on your back, but it can also be done sitting, if required.

1. Place the hands over your lower abdomen and begin to breathe. Imagine that you are inhaling into your lower belly. You may need to relax a bit around your belly. Have the feeling of letting go of the tension that you hold in and around your waistband.

2. As you breathe in, feel your belly expand under your hands, a bit like a balloon inflating. As you exhale, feel your belly release, like a balloon deflating.

3. As you focus on this sensation, allow the breath naturally to deepen and lengthen. To begin with, you may need to deliberately make your belly rise and fall, but as you get used to this breath, it will start to feel more natural.

Three-Part Breath

The Three-Part Breath (yogic breath) brings us into awareness of our full breathing capacity. When someone is stressed, it is quite common for them to breathe in a very shallow way or to hold their breath. Some people may also feel breathless because of reduced lung capacity or low blood count. The full yogic breath allows people to access the full extent of the breath that is available to them and to fully oxygenate their body.

You can do this exercise sitting or, if it's comfortable for you, lying down.

1. Begin with your hands over your lower abdomen. Imagine you are inhaling into your lower belly. Breathe like this for a few breaths. Feel your abdomen expand under your hands as you inhale, as if you are inflating a balloon.

2. Next, move your hands on to the sides of your ribs and begin to feel your ribs expanding with your breath. Breathe like this for a few breaths.

3. Now move your hands on to your upper chest, just under your collar bones, so you can feel your chest expanding with your breath. Breathe like this for a few breaths.

4. You can now put the Three-Part Breath together. Inhale into your abdomen, then your ribs, then your chest. Exhale in reverse order, first from your chest, then your ribs, then your lower belly. Breathe smoothly. Continue breathing in and out very deeply for one to two minutes to start.

5. If you enjoy this practice you can work up to five minutes. Make the in-breath and out-breath equal and as long and sustained as you can, but keep it easy.

▧ QUESTIONS FOR REFLECTION

What aspects of someone's condition or treatment might you need to take into account when offering these practices? What might make the practice difficult for them? How might you adapt it? Would it be appropriate at all?

Pranayama

We don't tend to go deeply into the practices of Pranayama in modern postural yoga. And there is probably a good reason for that. Very few modern teachers are trained in the depth and subtleties of Pranayama, never mind its potentially potent effects. You just have to Google 'Is Pranayama dangerous?' for some insight into why this might be the case.

In Yoga for Cancer, we are even more circumspect. Pranayama – by its very definition – involves practices that work with the vital energy flow in the body. One of the essential components of many Pranayama practices is Kumbhaka, or breath retention. I don't tend to use breath retention in this work, because it can be quite stressful for someone whose system is already taxed. There may be exceptions – for example, if someone already has a developed practice of yoga or breathing. In this case, my oft-repeated adage 'it depends' comes back into play.

The Pranayama we look at here are tempered versions of the classical exercises, used for their specific benefits. I do not practise the more rigorous exercises such as Kapalabhati or Bhastrika. These exercises are too strong for most inexperienced practitioners and certainly for those whose system is weakened by illness or treatment.

I have also made the – possibly controversial – decision to not include Nadi Shodhana Pranayama (Alternate Nostril Breathing, ANB) despite the fact that it is a go-to for many yoga practitioners who want a calming practice. This is not to say that you must not do ANB. We are taught that ANB helps to calm the mind and the nervous system, and this is true – if the practice is sustained over time, seasoned yoga practitioners find it very beneficial. However, I have found that the coordination required can be difficult for a person who is feeling particularly tired or who is experiencing 'chemo-brain'. If the person can't get the hang of it, the stress of trying can outweigh the benefits. Evidence seems to suggest that a long-term practice of ANB is beneficial, but it doesn't really help in the short term.[43] If your student already has a yoga practice, then it is definitely worth trying.

In truth, it is unlikely that you will spend much time teaching full-on Pranayama to people living with cancer. My experience has been that simply giving people encouragement to breathe normally – or indeed, to breathe at all – is often enough.

Ujjayi (victorious breath)

Ujjayi is a practice for slowing the breath, and there is some evidence that breathing techniques that slow down the air flow, as well as having a direct effect on the parasympathetic response, can help to restore vagal tone (as we saw in Chapter Two), and thus additionally reduce the effects of stress.

Ujjayi is a strange practice in yoga. In some practices – such as Ashtanga Vinyasa – its use is encouraged throughout the Asana practice, and in other practices it is only used as a (fairly) advanced Pranayama practice. My own thoughts are mixed. I feel its use is very much dependent on the individual person's energy. Traditionally Ujjayi is a heating practice, and is therefore not always appropriate during cancer treatment that might cause hot flushes. If someone is otherwise hot, for example, with a fever or high blood pressure, Ujjayi may not be useful. It may also aggravate a sore or dry throat. Therefore, although Ujjayi is a potentially very potent stress-reducing practice, it can be counterproductive.

I really play it by ear, and if the person would really benefit from using it, then I use it. If the person has the type of personality that might get hung up on doing it 'right' or if they seem to be using force to achieve the Ujjayi sound, I will avoid it. If, however, we can achieve a gentle Ujjayi without force, it can be very useful.

1. Sit in a comfortable position. Breathe gently through your nostrils and simply watch your breath for a while, without changing it in any way.

2. Now begin to breathe gently through your mouth. Feel the air passing over the back of your throat. Then on your exhalation very slightly constrict the back of your throat, making a sighing 'hahhh' sound as you exhale. (Tip: Imagine the way you steam up your glasses to clean them.)

3. As you become comfortable with your exhalation, maintain the slight constriction of the throat on your inhalation as

well. Your breath will make the sighing sound, softly moving in and out, like the sound of the sea.

4. When you are comfortable making the Ujjayi sound with your mouth open, you can gently close your mouth and begin breathing only through your nose. Keep the same constriction in your throat as you did when your mouth was open. You will continue to hear the sighing sound as you breathe through your nose. Direct the breath to travel over the back of your throat. Keep your mouth closed but relaxed.

5. Focus on the sound of your breath. You can practise breath awareness using the Ujjayi breath. As with all of the breathing practices, stop if you feel dizzy. Keep it easy and comfortable. You can continue for a few minutes or as long as it feels comfortable.

Bhramari (humming (bee) breath)

I LOVE Bhramari, for all sorts of reasons! Because it involves slowing the breath down, it is an incredibly calming and balancing Pranayama. It also involves making sound, which has additional benefits, including influencing heart rate variability.[44] Because it involves closing off the ears, so that you hear the sound inside your own head, the sound has the effect of reducing unwanted thoughts, and seems to have an energizing, awakening effect, a bit like a rinse for the brain. Also, because it is fun, people are often open to trying it when they might not be so open to mantras or chanting. Research has also shown that humming increases the level of the chemical nitric oxide that is potentially beneficial for sinus health,[45] essentially helping us to breathe more easily.

1. Sit comfortably with your eyes closed.

2. Place your thumbs on the cartilage between your cheek and ear. Using your thumb tip, close the opening of your ear by gently pressing the cartilage. Place your index and middle fingers *gently* over your eyes with the tips of your fingers between your inner eye and the bridge of your nose. Do not

press down on your eyes. Place the tip of your ring finger gently above your nostrils and your little fingers just above your upper lip.

3. Inhale through your nose and as you exhale, make a humming sound (like a bee!). Do a few rounds like this, maybe six to nine times.

4. Release your hands, and let your breathing return to normal. Notice the effects of the practice. Repeat if it feels appropriate.

Practice Bhramari as often as you can! Trying to force the breath, or breathing out for longer than feels comfortable, will just make you more stressed, so take it easy, and keep it relaxed.

▨ QUESTION FOR REFLECTION
Why do you think it may not be a good idea to teach exercises like Kapalabhati or Bhastrika to people undergoing treatment for cancer?

Golden Thread Breath
Panic is not uncommon when someone is under extreme stress. And the diagnosis and treatment of a life-threatening illness is a very stressful event. Often the treatments are traumatic. Panic can manifest in a number of ways and it can arise in reaction to a situation, or seemingly out of the blue. I have encountered this in hospital work when people have to go through difficult procedures that are painful, isolating or claustrophobic. And having an accessible and quick-acting breathing method up my sleeve was very helpful.

One of the most profound practices I have encountered to alleviate panic attacks and the effects of shallow breathing is the Golden Thread Breath. Many people learn this on their pregnancy yoga training as it is a fantastic preparation for the kind of breathing that is beneficial during labour. But it also has a wonderful effect on overcoming the hyperventilation that often accompanies panic.

The Golden Thread Breath involves exhaling with your mouth very slightly open and extending the length of the exhale. It is a beautifully calming exercise, and the visualization helps gently to extend the exhalation without strain.

1. Sit comfortably with your eyes closed and establish a comfortable breath, breathing in and out of your nose.

2. After a few breaths, part your lips and teeth slightly, as though you are holding a petal or a tiny straw between them, continuing to breathe in through your nose but allowing the out-breath to pass through your lips and teeth. Your face, lips and breath are soft, and your exhalation will become longer as it almost trickles from between your lips.

3. As you exhale, visualize the breath as a fine golden thread that spins from between your lips and out into the room. The longer the breath becomes, the further you can visualize the golden thread spinning into the distance.

If you find it hard to visualize, or the visualization feels weird (it doesn't work for everyone!) you can focus on the sensation or the gentle sound of your breath, or just the concept of the breath extending out into space.

Breathlessness

Some people will have conditions – either pre-existing or related to their cancer or treatment – which will affect the quality of their breathing.

Things that can cause breathlessness include:

- Cancer that affects the lungs.

- Smoking.

- Low levels of red blood cells (anaemia).

- Fluid in the lungs or stomach.

- A chest infection.

- COPD (chronic obstructive pulmonary disease).

- Muscle weakness.

- Blood clots.

- Pain.

- Anxiety.

- Some cancer treatments.

You might encounter someone who feels that they are struggling to breathe, or who has to be treated with oxygen, in which case your gentle presence, encouraging easy breath awareness, will be very helpful. Depending on the severity, my advice is to avoid any special techniques or attempting to instruct the person on 'how' to breath, and to practise simple breath awareness. A focus on the space available for the breath might be helpful, rather than focusing on the difficulty.

Attending to your own breath
This scenario, where someone is really struggling to breathe, can have quote a strong somatic response in your own body, and might make you feel panicky. Focus on slow, mindful breathing in your own body. Even this practice can have an effect on the person you are with.

Paradoxical breathing
You may encounter someone whose belly and chest do the opposite of what you would expect on inhalation and exhalation, that is, instead of expanding on the inhalation they contract and expand on the exhalation. You are most likely to encounter this when someone has a medical condition that is affecting their breathing.

Conditions that might cause a paradoxical breathing pattern are:

- Injury to the chest.

- Neurological problems.

- Electrolyte or hormone imbalance.

- Muscle dysfunction.

- Upper airway blockage.

- Asthma.

- Sleep apnoea.

Hopefully, if you have taken a full medical history, you will know if the person has any particular medical issues. You can try and work on breathing techniques with them, but if it doesn't work, don't cause them any stress by forcing the issue. Simply work on slow gentle breathing and breath awareness. I would not work on any more complex breathing techniques with this person just yet.

■ QUESTION FOR REFLECTION
What modifications to a yoga practice might you consider offering to someone experiencing breathlessness? You might wish to look at resources on breathlessness from the Roy Castle Lung Cancer Foundation,[46] Macmillan[47] and the British Lung Foundation[48] (see 'Resources to Inform Your Research' at the end of the book).

Practical self-help
This section offers some additional resources that you can offer to people for practical self-help in addition to the personalized yoga practices that you give them:

- 'Soften, soothe and allow' helps with pain and/or nausea.

- 'Soothing self-touch' can also help with pain, or to bring calm.

- 'Abdominal self-massage' can help relieve constipation or tummy ache.

- And 'Coping with hiccups' does what it says on the tin!

Soften, soothe and allow

1. Find a comfortable position and close your eyes.

2. Place your hand over your heart for a few moments. Check in with yourself. Feel yourself present (on the bed/floor/chair), and allow yourself to be fully supported, held and safe. Take three deep breaths. Inhaling deeply and then

sighing the breath out. Bring your awareness to your body and how it feels. Notice your body as a whole. Scan your body from head to toe, stopping where you feel the sensation of pain, nausea or discomfort most acutely. In your mind, move gently towards that spot. Without wishing the sensation away, simply incline towards it, notice it.

3. Soften into that place in your body. Try and allow the muscles to become soft without trying to make it happen. Just let it happen, like applying a gentle heat to sore muscles. You are not trying to make the sensation go away – just let it be, but let it soften. Begin by softening around the edges, allowing the pain/nausea/discomfort to soften from the outside in. No rush. You might wish to repeat, mentally, the word 'soften...'

4. Soothe yourself. Put your hand over the area that is uncomfortable and feel your body breathe. You might find that words of self-comfort arise, or you can allow feelings of love and compassion to be directed from your hand into the area that needs to be soothed. It might feel soothing to attend to your body as if it was your child. You might wish to repeat, mentally, the word 'soothe...'

5. Allow the remaining discomfort to be there. Do not try and make the feeling go away. Simply allow the discomfort to come and go, like clouds across the sky. You might wish to repeat, mentally, the word 'allow'. As you stay with the sensations that arise, you can repeat the mantra 'Soften, soothe and allow'.

Soothing self-touch

Human beings need touch. And the body responds to touch, even when it is our own. Touch activates the release of oxytocin, a hormone that – amongst other things – assists in reducing stress hormones. It releases when we touch, and are touched by, another human being, and even an animal (and the animal has a release of oxytocin too!).

1. Give yourself a hug. Offering touch to yourself can be as easy as giving yourself a hug. Try it. Wrap your arms across your chest and give yourself the kind of hug that feels soothing or real for you in this moment. It might feel a bit strange to begin with, but even so, it can have a genuinely soothing effect.

2. Heart soothe. Place a hand or hands over your heart and feel the warmth there. Allow yourself to be soothed like you would soothe a child. Sometimes I invite people to warm their hands first by rubbing them together to create heat.

3. Belly rub. Place your hands over your belly and feel the sensation of heat. As above, you may wish to warm your hands first. Then begin to make gentle circling motions over the belly with the palms of the hands. Note: If you have diarrhoea, or have had recent abdominal surgery, or you have a stoma, don't rub; just simply place your hands.

4. Explore gentle self-touch in other ways, for example holding your face in your hands, massaging your scalp, rubbing your arms. See what is soothing to you.

Abdominal self-massage

Abdominal self-massage can be a highly effective way to cope with symptoms such as bloating, wind, nausea, abdominal cramp or pain and constipation. It can also be a very effective self-soothing technique, in much the same way as a baby is soothed by having its tummy rubbed.

DO NOT carry out abdominal self-massage if you have any of the following:

- Bowel cancer, surgery, or obstruction.

- Recent abdominal surgery – i.e., the wounds are still healing.

- Acute diarrhoea.

- Acute or severe nausea caused by a tummy upset.

- A stoma (colostomy, ileostomy, feeding tube).

- A tumour site in your abdomen.

- Abdominal pain that is sudden, acute and accompanied by fever or nausea (pain that is usual and related to an existing condition can often be alleviated; please take advice from your medical team if in doubt).

1. Place a hand over your abdomen.

2. Then, using the flat of your hand/base of the fingers, circle gently in a clockwise direction, following the line of the ascending, transverse and descending colon. The amount of pressure depends on how it feels. Listen to your body's signals.

3. You can then go anti-clockwise for a little while – 6–12 rotations – before resuming your clockwise massage.

Coping with hiccups

There is a very simple yoga technique that you can try if you are experiencing hiccups as a side effect of treatment, or just in general! It involves using breathing and a posture for the neck, which in yoga we call Jalandhara Bandha, or the 'chin lock'. Before you do this, let's check on a few things:

- Have you got very high or low blood pressure just now? If so, then this practice is not for you at the moment.

- Do you have heart disease or glaucoma? Again, this practice is not suitable.

- Do you have prolapsed discs or crushed vertebrae in your neck? Have you had recent surgery on your neck or throat? If so, then you can do the breathing bit, but not the chin lock.

- Have you had abdominal surgery or fluid retention in your abdominal area? If so, then don't contract the abdomen too deeply when you breathe out. Do what feels comfortable.

- If you feel dizzy or lightheaded or nauseous at any point, then stop and breathe deeply.

- Don't strain or force anything. If it doesn't feel easy, don't do it.

1. Sit or stand with the spine long and the shoulders relaxed.

2. Breathe easily. Tune into your breathing, noticing how the body moves as you breathe. Notice how your belly moves, rising and falling like a balloon inflating or deflating. Focus on allowing your breath to lengthen. Even if you are hiccupping the whole time, just let the hiccups come, and continue to follow your breath. As the breath gets a little bit longer and deeper, you can begin to gently draw the belly in at the end of your exhalation, like a gentle little 'hug' for your tummy. Let this feel completely natural and not strained.

3. After a few breaths, exhale deeply until all the air is out and then HOLD your breath OUT. At the same time let your chin draw towards your throat. This should feel like you are deliberately giving yourself a double chin. Hold here for as long as it doesn't feel strained. When you feel ready to breathe in, release the chin first, and let the breath come in naturally.

4. You can repeat the whole process two or three times until there is relief. STOP if anything doesn't feel good.

Mantra

Mantra is at the more esoteric end of the Hatha Yoga spectrum for Western practitioners, and, other than the odd 'Om' chanted at the end of a class, is often left out. This is a shame, because Mantra forms a valuable element of practice. For people living with cancer, we can offer Mantra as an empowering addition to the more common practices that involve the breath and postures.

Mantra is about using sound for invocation, healing and devotion to enhance the flow of energies or to aid meditation. A Mantra really can be any sound, word or phrase that is repeated, with intention, either out loud or internally. However, in the yogic and other Eastern spiritual traditions, there are very specific sounds and verses that are considered to carry very powerful vibrations. In the ancient yogic language of Sanskrit, this does not just apply to the words that are being repeated, but to the very syllables contained within the words. Whether, as modern practitioners, we buy into this belief or not is about how we approach our own practice.

My own experience of working with Mantra has been quite profound. I have a personal Mantra that was given to me in India via an empowerment Puja. I have also practised a 40-day Mantra discipline – getting up at dawn to chant the same Mantra 108 times every day for 40 days. The outcome was not insignificant. I can't say why this happened. Perhaps simply setting the intention, and knowing how I wanted the Mantra to help me, gave me the outcome that I was looking for, simply by altering my attitude or behaviour. Or maybe the Mantra's power really worked. Who knows? What I do know is that for me, something worked!

Even if the only thing that is beneficial about chanting a Mantra is using the voice to release tension, that's great. There are specific Mantras that people can use if they want to influence a certain energy in their life, or to honour specific deities, to offer as a devotion or invocation to their yoga practice, or to simply mark the start and finish of a practice.

Should you use Mantra working with people living with cancer? Well, as always, it depends! If the person is open to using sound, or having you use sound with them, and it doesn't make them think they are being recruited for a cult, then absolutely. Yes. But bear in mind that for some people, it's maybe just a bit too 'out there', so tread slowly. They might be more open to you chanting, and them enjoying the vibration, than doing it themselves.

Bija Mantras

Bija, in Sanskrit, means seed. The seed Mantras are one-syllable sounds that make up other Mantras, but that can also be chanted on their own. The elements that are associated with the Chakras are considered to have their own Bija Mantras, or sounds, that can be used to bring awareness to the energy centres.

Each element and its corresponding Chakra has a sound that works with the quality of vibration associated with it.

I would tend to use the Bija Mantras if I am working on a particular aspect of energy with a person. And they are very accessible in that regard. So, you can have someone take their hands to rest on the area of the body that corresponds to the Chakra, and have them chant this sound with you. For example, if I am focusing on the heart or chest, then I might incorporate the Mantra 'Yam', which is associated with the element of air, and the Heart Chakra. I find that people start off feeling a little self-conscious, but they do get into it, and find it an empowering part of the practice that they can do themselves!

Muladhara, Root Chakra
Mantra – Lam; element – Earth.

Svadhisthana, Sacral Chakra
Mantra – Vam; element – Water.

Manipura, Solar Plexus Chakra
Mantra – Ram; element – Fire.

Anahata, Heart Chakra
Mantra – Yam; element – Air.

Visuddha, Throat Chakra
Mantra – Ham; element – Ether.

Ajna, Third Eye Chakra
Mantra – Aum/Om.

Sahasrara, Crown Chakra
Mantra – Silence.

Om or Aum

'Om' is the vibrational aspect of, well, everything. The Universe. Creator. All that is. We are mostly used to chanting it at the beginning and end of yoga classes. And it serves beautifully as an invocation to most things. It sets up the energy for the practice. In terms of accessibility, most people can cope with an 'Aum' without feeling too uncomfortable.

'SoHam' Mantra

The 'SoHam' Mantra is a beautiful one to use for meditation. This one is usually done inwardly, rather than as an external sound or chant, because essentially it is the sound of the breath.

'SoHam' translates as 'I AM THAT'. So that when the Mantra begins to flow, it creates the pattern of 'IAMTHATIAMTHATIAMTHA-TIAMTHAT'. It equates to the individual soul or consciousness being one with the universal consciousness.

Inhale 'So'; exhale 'Ham' (sounds like 'Hum'); inhale 'So'; exhale 'Ham', and so on.

'SoHam' is a beautiful way to connect deeply with the breath, and I have found that it can help people who are struggling with their breathing, or certainly with breathing deeply. The Mantra helps to focus on the breath, without the mechanics of the breath becoming so much of a barrier.

Mudra

Mudras are gestures or postures that are considered to seal or hold energy in the body. Often these are done as hand gestures, although they can also be done with the body. Mudra is a whole science in itself, and it is a very neglected part of Hatha Yoga these days as we focus more and more on just Asana. Mudras are considered to work by influencing the direction and flow of vital energy in the body in order to positively affect psychological, emotional or physical wellbeing. There are hundreds of Mudras, and different ones for different philosophical approaches. If you want to delve more deeply into Mudra, I highly recommend reading more. Some suggestions for books and resources are given at the end of the book.

The following Mudras are my suggestions for hand gestures that I have found helpful to use with people living with cancer. I exercise judgement about with whom I use them, as they are a little esoteric for some, but some people are very open to them. On a symbolic level, they can help people to remember to come to back to the way of feeling (still, relaxed, etc.) that they felt when they were doing the practice with you, a way of 'sealing' it into the body's memory, so to speak. You can use Mudras to accompany meditation, visualization or even Asana to set intention, or to focus on a particular mind state or energy.

Anjali Mudra, for connection and awareness

Anjali = a gesture of reverence, benediction, salutation (from Anj, to honour, celebrate).

1. Bring your palms together with the thumbs resting against your breast.

2. Press the hands firmly but evenly against each other. Bow your head slightly.

Practising Anjali Mudra is an excellent way to induce a meditative state of awareness. Start or finish your practice sitting in meditation in Anjali Mudra, or to focus, connect or centre during a practice.

Padma (Lotus) Mudra, to nourish the heart

1. The hands are held at heart centre. Bring the heels of the palms together, thumb tips and tips of the little fingers touching. Keep your knuckles separate and let your fingers blossom like the petals of a flower.

This can be a beautiful mudra to accompany Metta meditation or any work around love, compassion or healing.

Ganesha Mudra, for strength and courage

Ganesha = the elephant-headed God, son of Shiva and Parvati; Ganapathi: the remover of obstacles.

This Mudra also works with the Heart Chakra, but in a way that brings the benefits of strength, courage and tenacity.

1. Bring both hands in front of your chest and take the left hand with the palm facing outwards with the thumb pointing towards your solar plexus and your little finger pointing towards your collar bone.

2. Bend the four fingers of your left hand and clasp them with the four fingers of your right hand. In this position, your right palm should be facing towards your chest. Inhale deeply. On the exhale, try to pull both arms apart while keeping all eight fingers locked. Feel the stretch along your shoulders and chest.

3. Repeat three or six times.

4. Then swap the position of the hands, with your right palm facing outwards and the left palm facing inwards and repeat this process. Release all tension from the arms and bring them close to your chest so that your hands are touching your sternum. Sit in this position for as long as you like and focus on your breath.

This Mudra also works with the Heart Chakra, but in a way that brings the benefits of strength, courage and tenacity.

Prana Mudra, for energy and vitality
Prana = energy, life force.

1. Keep your eyes closed and focus on your breath.

2. Touch the tips of your ring finger and little finger to your thumb. The index and middle finger should be pointed straight. The arms are by the sides or resting on the legs.

Prana Mudra helps to make you feel energized when you are fatigued or depressed. It is also considered to be helpful for strengthening the immune system.

CHAPTER NINE

Svadhyaya

Studying myself,
I learn and reflect, and find
spiritual growth.

In this penultimate chapter, I centre the discussion around Svadhyaya, which translates as self-study. In a yoga practice, this refers specifically to the ways in which we examine our own thought processes and behaviours as we follow the yogic path. In the context of our study of Yoga for Cancer, it also has this meaning, but here, I relate it to the ways in which we create a healthy, reflective and accountable professional teaching practice. This is important, I believe, for anyone who undertakes a role of teaching, guiding or influencing. This is particularly important when working with a vulnerable population.

Specifically, I look at reflective practice, supervision and mentoring as practices or methods in which you can gain deeper insight, support and direction with your ongoing teaching journey. Reflective practice and supervision are possibly less familiar to you than the concept of mentoring, unless you are already in a profession, such as nursing, social work or psychotherapy, where these practices are commonplace.

Reflective practice

You may have picked up by now that I have a little bee in my bonnet about professionalism and accountability in yoga teaching. It's one of the reasons I have written this book. And it's one of the reasons that throughout, you have been given regular opportunities to reflect on the material and consider your own responses, feelings, attitudes and practices. This is a form of reflective practice, taking a regular review of yourself, your practice and anything that crops up in your teaching. It is an opportunity for personal accountability and can – if you are open to it – provide many opportunities for self-development and growth as a teacher.

It is not quite the same as simply reflecting. As the name suggests, it is an active practice that requires a more practical engagement. Reflective practice is commonly taught to and required of teachers in education, nurses, social workers, etc., and there are several academic models of reflective practice that you might like to research.

One such model that you might find useful is the work of Gibbs (1988),[49] which can be summarized as follows:

1. Description of what happened.

2. Explore how you feel about it.

3. What went well? What needs improvement or development?

4. Why was this, do you think? What might help?

5. What do I need to do/learn/find out about?

6. How will I put this into action?

Of course, this works cyclically. When you get to 6, you go back to 1.

If I were to apply this to a practical example, it might look like this:

1. One of the members of my Yoga for Cancer class told me today that he has received a stage 4 diagnosis (terminal).

2. I didn't know what to say. I feel guilty that I didn't know what to say. I was upset too, as I am very fond of him and I was worried about displaying my own emotion.

3. I managed to get through the class today but I felt rattled and I am sure it showed. I don't think I gave enough time for

the class to process the information. I wasn't sure if that was appropriate.

4. It was unexpected. Or maybe it wasn't. I don't know. I am worried that I am out of my depth. What if I can't handle it?

5. Maybe I need to talk to someone who is more experienced in this sort of thing? I think I will go back and read *Being with Dying* – I remember it was really helpful in learning to be with difficult emotions.

6. I will book a mentoring or supervision session. I will re-read *Being with Dying* and look up other resources around compassionate presence. I will remember that my own practice is really important.

Practice journal

My students are not required to buy many books, but one that is on the required 'reading list' is a blank journal or notebook, which comes along with the strong invitation to keep a daily practice journal. This is a useful thing for anyone with an active practice, and certainly for anyone who chooses to teach that practice. For someone who chooses to specialize in working with people who are in any way vulnerable, such as people living with cancer, then I would suggest that it is essential.

Supervision

Clinical or professional supervision is common in professions such as psychotherapy and counselling, but it is not standard in complementary therapies or in yoga. And yet, the emotional impact of working with people, and especially people with additional needs, can be considerable. It is not always appropriate for you to offload on your nearest and dearest. There are issues of confidentiality for one thing, but also it can be damaging to personal relationships constantly to bring this stuff home.

Supervision need not be as formal as it sounds, but my belief is that it is essential if you are working in a therapeutic role. Another senior yoga teacher or therapist – someone who has a long-term practice – may be willing to offer this to you. This is also a valuable relationship if you encounter an area of practice that you are unsure about.

The Care Quality Commission (CQC) in the UK defines supervision as follows[50]:

> Professional supervision is […] where supervision is carried out by another member of the same profession or group. This can provide staff with the opportunity to:
>
> - Review professional standards.
>
> - Keep up to date with developments in their profession.
>
> - Identify professional training and continuing development needs.
>
> - Ensure that they are working within professional codes of conduct and boundaries.

QUESTIONS FOR REFLECTION

How might you benefit from having professional supervision?

Who in your network might be able to do this for you? (It should be someone with a mature practice, and ideally someone with experience in a supervision role.)

Mentoring

At first glance, mentoring and supervision might seem very similar, and in many respects they are. One of the key differences, however, is that supervision is essentially a space into which you bring those aspects of your practice that you know need the sounding board of a more experienced practitioner. The reflective practice model above is one such example.

Mentoring can certainly be supervision, but not always. It can take many forms – formal and informal – and it can be carried out by someone more experienced, by a peer, even by someone in an entirely different profession. It is a relationship that supports the mentee

– through encouragement, questioning, accountability, emotional cheerleading and simple presence – to support and develop themselves and their practice.

There are also mentoring groups for yoga teachers online as well as in the 'real world' that it might be worth accessing to use as a sounding board. Do always bear in mind all of the aspects of confidentiality that we discussed in Chapter Three, and be very mindful, if you join a mentoring group on social media, that not everyone in a group will hold to the same ethical principles as you do, so be measured and discerning about what you share.

I also highly recommend the book *The Yoga Teacher Mentor*[51] written by my friend and colleague Jess Glenny, which is a reflective journey through the various experiential aspects of being a yoga teacher.

CHAPTER TEN

Ishvara Pranhidana

I am in service
to something greater than self.
This is connection.

Ishvara Pranhidana may well be the most difficult of the Niyamas for a secular yoga audience to get their heads around. And for that reason, it is often overlooked. Ishvara in Sanskrit has many meanings, but in modern Hinduism, it more regularly refers to the idea of the personal nature of God, or indeed, a personal deity like Shiva. Patañjali defined Ishvara as the 'special self', and modern yoga practitioners often define it as the higher self, or spiritual self, true self, or whatever the individual relates to in terms of the spiritual aspect of themselves or of nature.

Pranhidana means to surrender or devote. As such, Ishvara Pranhidana invites us to surrender to, or devote our practice to God. In this context I offer another possibility, that it is to be in service to something greater than ourselves. For some this may well be God, for others, another sense of higher reality, and for yet others, this may mean service to the community, society or the greater good. This last focus is the one I have chosen for this chapter. Specifically I examine ways in which you can be in service to your students who are living through a diagnosis of cancer, to those you may seek to work in partnership with, and how you might choose to market your work from an ethical perspective.

Being of service to your students
Integrating into your existing classes

You may already be teaching people living with cancer in your regular classes, which is perhaps why you purchased this book. Or you may be in training as a yoga therapist or specialist teacher and using this book as a textbook. Either way, having worked your way through the material, you may have found that your style of teaching has changed. You might be feeling more compassionate, more aware of diverse needs and more deeply connected to people. And if that is the case, then this book has done its work. You may not choose to do any more with it, and that is fine. More than fine.

However, what I usually find when I lead my students through this process is that they inevitably feel much more confident and ready to welcome people with cancer – and indeed, people with other illnesses or disabilities – into their general classes, even when they were terrified of the idea at the beginning. It is only in part because they have more knowledge. Mostly, it is down to the awareness that they are equipped to welcome the person, to gently assist in modifying the practice, and to do all of this in the spirit of loving, compassionate presence.

Working one to one

Working privately or one to one with someone living with cancer is the ideal way to adapt the practice entirely to the needs of the person. It is also a deeply rewarding way to work. You may already be doing this with existing clients, and I hope that this book has given you more knowledge and more confidence to offer your clients the support that they need. I encourage you to consider additional training if you are going to offer Yoga for Cancer as a specialism. If you are not certified as a yoga therapist or as a Yoga for Cancer teacher, then please do make sure that this is clear to the people you work with. Being clear and upfront about your qualifications and experience is part of the ethical approach that underpins this book and my trainings.

The best and most successful approach I have found in my years doing this work is word of mouth. If you let it be known that you are offering this work, it is highly likely that people will find you, and tell other people about what you are doing.

Working in partnership

If you want to offer specialist classes for groups of people living with cancer, then you are going to have to do some networking. I am not going to pretend that this is an easy world to get into, but with a little tenacity, and a lot of integrity, you might just find yourself in a wonderful situation. Below are some ideas for organizations and groups you can approach or consider.

If the idea of networking makes you cringe – and I admit it does to me! – it is worthwhile remembering that it doesn't have to be about selling anything. It is about building relationships. And relationships are about trust. Just go and say hello.

Local hospital oncology centre or unit

Find the lead nurse or clinical nurse specialist and see if you can arrange a meeting. Each hospital specialism will probably have a lead or specialist nurse, for example, a breast care nurse. They might arrange to see you, but they are understandably very busy and not the easiest people to get hold of. Rightly, their first priority is the patients. They might give out your information to patients if they think it is going to be helpful, so it's worth a shot.

Local cancer support groups

These are always a useful source of local contact, although they don't often have much money. They might be willing to fundraise, or tap into grant money for a specific project. You might also consider volunteering to do this on their behalf. Depending on the area in which you live, local businesses often want to be associated with donating to, or raising funds for, local charities, so it is definitely worth pursuing, if fundraising is one of your skills or strengths.

Hospices

Hospices often offer yoga and complementary therapies – often as a day centre service to people in the community. Some hospices do recruit their complementary therapists as volunteers, though, and they may well expect the yoga to come free. But some do have a budget for activities.

GP surgeries or primary care facilities

Your local GP surgeries may offer to display your posters if not refer people to you. With the introduction of 'social prescribing' in the UK, some surgeries have link workers whose job it is to refer patients to community services, like yoga classes. If you have a good relationship with your GP practice, you might be able to persuade them to let you come and do a talk on the benefits of yoga. GPs are required to do continuing professional development (CPD), and such talks can be part of that.

Cancer centres

Some larger towns have cancer centres, such as those run in the UK by Maggie's, Macmillan and other local organizations. They do tend to have funding and often have a regular yoga class. If they already have a yoga teacher, they may be willing to give you the opportunity to cover or sub their classes when their yoga teacher is off sick or on holiday.

Cancer charities

Some of the larger cancer charities like Macmillan in the UK fund support groups as well as learning resources, information officers and nurses. They are usually a good source of reliable evidence-based information and support, and have good national and local presence. Contacting your local support officer or information centre might be a good place to start to find out what is going on in your area. You can access information online or at information points in your local library, health centre or hospital.

Cancer – specific charities
There is a wealth of cancer-specific charities from those that focus on the most common cancers, and others that focus on raising awareness about rarer, less well-known, cancers. The larger, well-resourced charities often have a programme of awareness raising or wellbeing events that may require your expertise. For example, when I was working with a large breast cancer charity, I often needed to recruit yoga teachers and therapists in a local area, and I would always prioritize those with additional awareness or training about cancer.

Local wellbeing businesses
Local businesses such as health food shops, complementary therapy clinics, hairdressers, beauty therapists, spas and gyms may all be a source of referral. People often go to these places when they have been unwell. They may happily refer clients to you, or you might be able to leave your business cards, flyers or posters.

Other local groups
Other local groups to consider that might not readily come to mind are the Women's Institute, church groups, Mother's Union, local elderly groups, community centres, exercise groups and various clubs. Everyone knows someone who has been touched by cancer.

Local authorities
Local authorities – district, county and city councils – often have pots of grant funding that you may be able to apply for to set up a class in your area. They are not always openly advertised, so it is definitely worth making some enquiries as to what might be available. Usually grants are made to local community groups, so it is more likely to be something you want to access on behalf of a local group, with the funding going to help pay for you, a venue, etc. Contact them directly to find out what is on offer. Yoga is certainly something I have seen funded on my local council's website.

Ethical marketing

If you are anything like me, the word 'marketing' is not exactly music to your ears. And I know that yoga teachers would rather be yoga teachers and not have to do any marketing. It doesn't need to be associated with the worst aspects of capitalism, making a profit, expanding your business, etc. You can do everything for free, if you wish. Marketing is just a way of getting your 'product' – in this case YOU – known by the people who would most benefit from it. You are offering a service, a gift that people really need, and they deserve to know about it.

Having said that, there is marketing, then there is marketing. We have spent the entirety of this book looking at the practices of Yoga for Cancer from within an ethical framework, and it would be remiss of me to leave marketing out of the need for ethical boundaries. How you promote what you do and what you say about the benefits of Yoga for Cancer should not be compromised for the sake of reaching a wider audience. At the root of ethical marketing is trust. My friend and colleague Steve Savides, who heads up The Global Trust Project,[52] says that basic elements of trust are integrity, benevolence and capability.

Here are some ways that you can ensure your marketing activities are ethical.

Tell the truth

As we covered in Chapter Two, be honest. Hopefully this goes without saying. Be clear and upfront about the benefits of Yoga for Cancer, your experience and your qualifications. This builds trust, and it makes sure that everyone you encounter knows that you work with integrity.

Make your work affordable

One of the more concerning aspects of the wellbeing 'industry' is that only people who can afford it can access complementary therapies. My suggestion is to offer a sliding scale for fees. Charge the normal rate for classes for those who can afford to pay, and charge less for those who can't. Perhaps even offer free spaces, or community spaces. Often people will donate extra money if they know that they are supporting someone who can't afford to pay.

Support other local enterprises

Your local area will have a number of businesses, community groups and charities that you can build relationships with that are of mutual support and benefit. This might be as simple as renting the local community hall or promoting the local yoga studio on your website.

Work in partnership with other yoga teachers

Competition is not a healthy way to generate trust. Ethical marketing is about collaboration, communication and working in a community. Try not to see yourself in competition with other yoga teachers. Reach out to them and see what you can do to support one another. Build relationships, spark friendships, build trust.

Use people's personal data responsibly

Don't email too often or send unsolicited communications. Absolutely abide by the GDPR guidelines. If people feel that they can trust you not to send them stuff they don't want, or too often, this will help them trust you and your offering.

Use social media responsibly

The things that you post on social media reflect on you as a professional. I probably don't need to say much more than that.

Use images ethically

Ensure that the images you use on social media like Facebook and Instagram are your own, or are copyright free. Credit other people's work. Make sure that any images you use of yourself in marketing are appropriate. For example, you doing a handstand on the beach in Goa wearing only a swimsuit is probably not the best choice to market a Yoga for Cancer class. Keep it tasteful, relevant and accessible.

■ QUESTION FOR REFLECTION

What organizations, groups or facilities do you have in your local area that it might be useful for you to start building relationships with?

Case Studies

The following case studies are hybrid scenarios based on the many people I have encountered in my years of work with people living with cancer. They are not based on any one individual's experience.

In each case, you might find it useful to consider developing a yoga practice that focuses on their specific needs, both in a one-to-one scenario and if you were to invite this person into a group class. What specific practices might you offer? What modifications would you need to employ? What props and supports would you use? Think about all of the practices that we have discussed, and the personal qualities and ethical values in which this exploration has been centred.

Margaret

Margaret is in her early forties and has ovarian cancer which has metastasized and has spread to other organs in her abdomen and pelvis. She had a hysterectomy and oophorectomy (removal of the ovaries), and this has brought on an early menopause. She is receiving chemotherapy as a palliative measure to try to slow the progress of the disease. The tumours in her abdomen are quite large, which she can 'feel'. She is – perhaps understandably – very down about her prognosis.

Daniel

Daniel is in his early fifties and is used to being very fit and active, He goes to the gym regularly. A couple of months ago he developed a cough, accompanied by severe back pain. He was diagnosed with lung cancer in his right lung. Daniel is currently receiving radiotherapy to try to reduce the size of the tumour in his lung before surgery. This is making him feel very fatigued. He feels frustrated that he is no longer able to the same physical activity that he is used to.

Maeve

Maeve is in her early sixties and is recovering from bowel cancer that was diagnosed just over a year ago. Maeve received chemotherapy and surgery. She had part of the bowel removed and now has an ileostomy. She has also been advised to eat as much as possible to build her up after significant weight loss, but has to avoid high fibre foods, as her digestive system can't cope with those right now.

Resources to Inform Your Research

Bowel Cancer UK: www.bowelcanceruk.org.uk

British Lung Foundation: www.blf.org.uk

Cancer Research UK: www.cancerresearchuk.org

Macmillan: www.macmillan.org.uk

Ovarian Cancer Action: https://ovarian.org.uk

Roy Castle Lung Cancer Foundation: www.roycastle.org

Stomawise: www.stomawise.co.uk

Target Ovarian Cancer: www.targetovariancancer.org.uk

Endings and Next Steps

Thank you for reaching the end of this book, and for joining me on this deep, ethically inspired journey of heart, body and mind. If you have worked your way systematically through the book, you might find yourself at a place where you feel ready to offer yoga to people living with cancer. You might already be doing this, and the book has helped you to feel more resourced and confident. It is also possible that it has opened up many more questions for you, which wouldn't surprise me. One of the things that I am aware of, the older I get and the more I work with yoga, is that the more I know, the more I am aware of what I don't know!

I highly recommend additional training if you are relatively new to yoga teaching and/or if you haven't done any therapeutic yoga training before.

You can read about my own work in Yoga for Cancer at www.my-healingspace.org.uk

I also offer my Healing Space Yoga for Cancer training as an online modular course at https://healing-space.teachable.com

I teach a Yoga for Cancer training course for yoga teachers via Yoga-campus. Their headquarters are in London, but they offer in person trainings in other UK locations and increasingly, online and blended learning options for international students. They also offer excellent CPD for more experienced teachers. They offer a Yoga Therapy Diploma course and specialist courses and short workshops on a wide range of topics, and cover therapeutic yoga for a wide range of health conditions including chronic fatigue/ME and mental health. Yogacampus work with highly skilled and experienced teachers who are all experts in their field: www.yogacampus.com

I have mentioned the Yoga Nidra Network before, but I will plug them again for their excellent, ethically sound trainings and generous free resources: www.yoganidranetwork.org

I highly recommend the work of Dr Theodora Wildcroft who has done extensive research and published on the topic of 'Post-Lineage Yoga' and has a special interest in trauma-informed yoga spaces. She offers workshops, talks and trainings on the subject: www.wildyoga.co.uk

Jess Glenny is a London-based teacher and yoga therapist who specializes in trauma, hypermobility and yoga teacher mentoring. She offers regular workshops and one-to-one and group mentoring for teachers: www.embodyyogadance.co.uk

Further Reading

Ashley-Farrand, T. (2000) *Healing Mantras*. Nevada City, CA: Gateway.

Glenny, J. (2020) *The Yoga Teacher Mentor*. London and Philadelphia, PA: Singing Dragon.

Halifax, J. (2014) *Being with Dying: Cultivating Compassion and Fearlessness in the Presence of Death*. Boston, MA: Shambhala.

Halifax, J. (2019) *Standing at the Edge: Finding Freedom Where Fear and Courage Meet*. New York: Flatiron Books.

Hirschi, G. (2000) *Mudras: Yoga in Your Hands*. York Beach, ME: Samuel Weiser.

Kwok, J. (2017) *Yoga for Breast Cancer Survivors and Patients*.

Maté, G. (2019) *When the Body Says No: The Cost of Hidden Stress*. London: Vermilion.

Nischala, J.D. (2000) *The Healing Path of Yoga: Time-honored Wisdom and Scientifically Proven Methods that Alleviate Stress, Open Your Heart, and Enrich Your Life*. New York: Three Rivers Press.

Nouwen, H.J.M. (2014) *The Wounded Healer: Ministry in Contemporary Society*. London: Darton, Longman & Todd.

O'Donohue, J. (2004) *Divine Beauty: The Invisible Embrace*. London: Bantam Press.

O'Donohue, J. (2008) *Benedictus: A Book of Blessings*. Transworld Ireland.

Patañjali (2002) *Yoga Sutras of Patañjali*. Translated by Mukunda Stiles. Boston, MA: Weiser Books.

Prabhavananda, S. and Isherwood, C. (2018) *How to Know God: The Yoga Aphorisms of Patañjali*. London: Routledge.

Remski, M.D. (2019) *Practice and All Is Coming: Abuse, Cult Dynamics, and Healing in Yoga and Beyond*. Rangiora, New Zealand: Embodied Wisdom Publishing.

Sontag, S. (2002) *Illness as Metaphor*. London: Penguin Books.

Stevens, A. (2015) *Archetype Revisited: An Updated Natural History of the Self*. London: Routledge, Taylor & Francis Group.

Stiles, M. (2010) *Ayurvedic Yoga Therapy*. Twin Lakes, WI: Lotus Press.

Wildcroft, T. (2020) *Post-Lineage Yoga: From Guru to #metoo*. Sheffield: Equinox Publishing Ltd.

Endnotes

1   Patañjali (2002) *Yoga Sutras of Patañjali*. Translated by Mukunda Stiles. Boston, MA: Weiser Books.
2   Halifax, J. (2014) *Being with Dying: Cultivating Compassion and Fearlessness in the Presence of Death*. Boston, MA: Shambhala.
3   ONS (Office for National Statistics) (2013) 'What are the top causes of death by age and gender?' Available at: https://webarchive.nationalarchives.gov.uk/20160105221750/http://www.ons.gov.uk/ons/rel/vsob1/mortality-statistics--deaths-registered-in-england-and-wales--series-dr-/2012/sty-causes-of-death.html [accessed 13 June 2020].
4   Cancer Research UK (2017) 'What is cancer?' Available at: www.cancerresearchuk.org/about-cancer/what-is-cancer [accessed 11 August 2020].
5   World Cancer Research Fund (2018) 'Worldwide cancer data: Global cancer statistics for the most common cancers.' 6 August. Available at: www.wcrf.org/dietand-cancer/cancer-trends/worldwide-cancer-data#:~:text=Lung%20and%20breast%20cancers%20were [accessed 11 August 2020].
6   Granger, K. (2014) 'Having cancer is not a fight or a battle.' *The Guardian*, 25 April. Available at: www.theguardian.com/society/2014/apr/25/having-cancer-not-fight-or-battle [accessed 25 April 2019].
7   Gajewsky, M. (2015) 'May I take your metaphor? – how we talk about cancer.' Cancer Research UK – Science Blog, 25 September. Available at: https://scienceblog.cancer-researchuk.org/2015/09/28/may-i-take-your-metaphor-how-we-talk-about-cancer/ [accessed 13 June 2020].
8   Chandwani, K.D., G. Perkins, H.R. Nagendra, N.V. Raghuram, and others (2014) 'Randomized, controlled trial of yoga in women with breast cancer undergoing radiotherapy.' *Journal of Clinical Oncology 32*(10), 1058–1065. Available at: https://doi.org/10.1200/jco.2012.48.2752 [accessed 11 August 2020].
9   Green McDonald, P., M. O'Connell and S.K. Lutgendorf (2013) 'Psychoneuroimmunology and cancer: A decade of discovery, paradigm shifts, and methodological innovations.' *Brain, Behavior, and Immunity 30*, S1–9. Available at: https://doi.org/10.1016/j.bbi.2013.01.003 [accessed 13 August 2020].
10 Maté, G. (2019) *When the Body Says No: The Cost of Hidden Stress*. London: Vermilion.
11 Agarwal, R.P. and A. Maroko-Afek (2018) 'Yoga into cancer care: A review of the evidence-based research.' *International Journal of Yoga 11*(1), 3–29. Medknow Publications and Media Pvt Ltd. Available at: https://pubmed.ncbi.nlm.nih.gov/29343927/?

12 Kiecolt-Glaser, J.K., J.M. Bennett, R. Andridge, J. Peng, and others (2014) 'Yoga's impact on inflammation, mood, and fatigue in breast cancer survivors: A randomized controlled trial.' *Journal of Clinical Oncology 32*(10), 1040–1049. Available at: https://doi.org/10.1200/jco.2013.51.8860 [accessed 13 August 2020].

13 Bower, J.E., G. Greendale, A.D. Crosswell, D. Garet, and others (2014) 'Yoga reduces inflammatory signaling in fatigued breast cancer survivors: A randomized controlled trial.' *Psychoneuroendocrinology 43*, 20–29. Available at: https://doi.org/10.1016/j.psyneuen.2014.01.019 [accessed 13 August 2020].

14 See https://pubmed.ncbi.nlm.nih.gov/

15 pH is the scientific measure of acidity or alkalinity in a solution. A pH of 7 is neutral. The higher the value, the more alkaline the solution is. The pH of the blood is tightly regulated between 7.35 and 7.45.

16 The Society of Analytical Psychology (no date) 'Home.' Jungian Psychology. Available at: www.thesap.org.uk/ [accessed 16 June 2020].

17 Nouwen, H.J.M. (2014) *The Wounded Healer: Ministry in Contemporary Society.* London: Darton, Longman & Todd.

18 GMC (General Medical Council) (2018) 'Disclosing patients' personal information: A framework.' Available at: www.gmc-uk.org/ethical-guidance/ethical-guidance-for-doctors/confidentiality/disclosing-patients-personal-information-a-framework [accessed 13 August 2020].

19 ICO (Information Commissioner's Office) (2019) 'Guide to the General Data Protection Regulation (GDPR).' Available at: https://ico.org.uk/for-organisations/guide-to-data-protection/guide-to-the-general-data-protection-regulation-gdpr/ [accessed 13 August 2020].

20 See www.nhs.uk/conditions/colostomy/

21 www.bacp.co.uk/

22 Macmillan Cancer Support (no date) 'Inclusion resources and publications – What we do.' Available at: www.macmillan.org.uk/about-us/what-we-do/how-we-work/inclusion/resources-and-publications.html#268633 [accessed 16 June 2020].

23 Equality and Human Rights Commission (2010) 'Protected characteristics.' Available at: www.equalityhumanrights.com/en/equality-act/protected-characteristics [accessed 13 August 2020].

24 Halifax, J. (2019) *Standing at the Edge: Finding Freedom Where Fear and Courage Meet.* New York: Flatiron Books.

25 Mills, J. (no date) 'Om Sahana Vavatu.' Available at: https://soundcloud.com/jude-mills/om-sahana-vavatu/s-y9iSUBiDlgN [accessed 16 June 2020].

26 Radha, Swami Sivananda (2010) *The Divine Light Invocation.* Kootenay Bay, BC: Timeless Books.

27 www.youtube.com/user/yasodharaashram

28 Halifax, J. (2014) *Being with Dying: Cultivating Compassion and Fearlessness in the Presence of Death.* Boston, MA: Shambhala.

29 www.johnodonohue.com

30 https://maryoliver.beacon.org/

31 Whyte, D. (no date) 'David Whyte & Many Rivers.' Available at: www.davidwhyte.com/ [accessed 30 June 2020].

32 Poetry Chaikhana (no date) 'Sacred Poetry from Around the World.' Available at: www.poetry-chaikhana.com/ [accessed 30 June 2020].

33 Stiles, M. (2010) *Ayurvedic Yoga Therapy.* Twin Lakes, WI: Lotus Press.

34 Gerritsen, R.J.S. and G.P.H. Band (2018) 'Breath of life: The respiratory vagal stimu-lation model of contemplative activity.' *Frontiers in Human Neuroscience 12.* Available at: https://doi.org/10.3389/fnhum.2018.00397 [accessed 13 August 2020].

35 Germer, C. (2019) 'Mindful Self-Compassion and Psychotherapy.' Available at: https://chrisgermer.com/ [accessed 13 August 2020].

36 Neff, K. (2015) 'Self-Compassion.' Available at: https://self-compassion.org/ [ac-cessed 13 August 2020].

37 Yoga Nidra Network (no date) 'Supporting Your Practice of Yoga Nidra.' Available at: www.yoganidranetwork.org [accessed 13 June 2020].

38 Total Yoga Nidra (no date) 'Total Yoga Nidra Teacher and Facilitator Training.' Avail-able at: www.yoganidranetwork.org/total-yoga-nidra-teacher-and-facilitator-train-ing [accessed 14 August 2020].

39 Prostate Cancer UK (no date) 'Surgery.' Available at: https://prostatecanceruk.org/prostate-information/treatments/surgery [accessed 1 July 2020].

40 Colostomy UK (no date) 'Colostomy UK – A UK Charity Supporting People with a Stoma.' Available at: www.colostomyuk.org [accessed 17 August 2020].

41 Macmillan (no date) 'What is a stoma?' Available at: www.macmillan.org.uk/cancer-in-formation-and-support/bowel-cancer/what-is-a-stoma [accessed 17 August 2020].

42 Breast Cancer Now (2019) 'Breast Cancer Research and Care Charity.' Available at: https://breastcancernow.org [accessed 17 August 2020].

43 Subramanian, R.K., P.R. Devaki and P. Salkumar (2016) 'Alternate nostril breath-ing at different rates and its influence on heart rate variability in non practition-ers of yoga.' *Journal of Clinical and Diagnostic Research.* Available at: https://doi.org/10.7860/jcdr/2016/15287.7094 [accessed 17 August 2020].

44 Sujan, M.U., K.A. Deepika, S. Mulakur, A.P. John, N.M. Babina and T.N. Sathyaprabha (2015) 'Effect of Bhramari Pranayama (humming bee breath) on heart rate variability and hemodynamic – A pilot study.' *Autonomic Neuroscience 192,* 82. Available at: https://doi.org/10.1016/j.autneu.2015.07.093 [accessed 17 August 2020].

45 Granqvist, S., J. Sundberg, J.O. Lundberg and E. Weitzberg (2006) 'Paranasal sinus ventilation by humming.' *The Journal of the Acoustical Society of America 119*(5), 2611–2617. Available at: https://doi.org/10.1121/1.2188887 [accessed 17 August 2020].

46 Roy Castle Lung Cancer Foundation (2014) 'Lung Cancer – Breathlessness.' Available at: www.youtube.com/watch?v=DcNQbbm9zXw [accessed 13 June 2020].

47 Macmillan (no date) 'Breathlessness.' Available at: www.macmillan.org.uk/cancer-in-formation-and-support/impacts-of-cancer/breathlessness [accessed 17 August 2020].

48 British Lung Foundation (2019) 'What can I do to manage my breathlessness?' Avail-able at: www.blf.org.uk/support-for-you/breathlessness/how-to-manage-breath-lessness [accessed 17 August 2020].

49 University of Edinburgh (2019) 'Gibbs' reflective cycle.' Available at: www.ed.ac.uk/reflection/reflectors-toolkit/reflecting-on-experience/gibbs-reflective-cycle [ac-cessed 17 August 2020].

50 CQC (Care Quality Commission) (2013) 'Supporting Information and Guidance: Supporting Effective Clinical Supervision.' *Registration under the Health and Social Care Act 2008.*

51 Glenny, J. (2020) *The Yoga Teacher Mentor.* London: Singing Dragon.

52 The Global Trust Project (no date) 'The Global Trust Project.' Available at: www.theglobaltrustproject.org/home [accessed 17 August 2020].

Index